FIGHT PCOS WITH DIET

A Comprehensive Insulin Resistance Diet Book for Women Having PCOS to Fight against Inflammation, Lose Weight and Improve Fertility

By

Sara Spencer

© Copyright 2020 by (Sara Spencer) - All rights reserved.

This document is geared towards providing exact and reliable information in regards to the topic and issue covered. The publication is sold with the idea that the publisher is not required to render accounting, officially permitted, or otherwise, qualified services. If advice is necessary, legal or professional, a practiced individual in the profession should be ordered.

- From a Declaration of Principles which was accepted and approved equally by a Committee of the American Bar Association and a Committee of Publishers and Associations.

In no way is it legal to reproduce, duplicate, or transmit any part of this document in either electronic means or in printed format. Recording of this publication is strictly prohibited and any storage of this document is not allowed unless with written permission from the publisher. All rights reserved.

The information provided herein is stated to be truthful and consistent, in that any liability, in terms of inattention or otherwise, by any usage or abuse of any policies, processes, or directions contained within is the solitary and utter responsibility of the recipient reader. Under no circumstances will any legal responsibility or blame be held against the publisher for any reparation, damages, or monetary loss due to the information herein, either directly or indirectly.

Respective authors own all copyrights not held by the publisher.

The information herein is offered for informational purposes solely, and is universal as so. The presentation of the information is without contract or any type of guarantee assurance.

The trademarks that are used are without any consent, and the publication of the trademark is without permission or backing by the trademark owner.

All trademarks and brands within this book are for clarifying purposes only and are the owned by the owners themselves, not affiliated with this document.

Table of Content

INTRODUCTION 6

CHAPTER 1: DIAGNOSING AND UNDERSTANDING PCOS 13

1.1 Effects of Diet on PCOS 15

1.2 Foods to Consume 21

1.3 Foods to Limit or Avoid 26

1.4 Other Lifestyle Changes To Consider 29

1.5 Research Findings Of nutritional Diet Plan for PCOS 32

1.6 What You Should Know About PCOS and Fertility 42

CHAPTER 2: PCOS AND PHYSICAL FITNESS 53

2.1 Shedding the Extra Load 54

2.2 Workout to Fight Pcos 63

CHAPTER 3: INSULIN RESISTANCE DIET AND PCOS .. 80

3.1 Coping with Insulin Resistance and Its Effects 83

3.2 The Glycemic Index and Diet 85

3.3 What Is Insulin Resistance Diet? 93

3.4 Other Advice for Healthy Eating 103

3.5 Taking Medications 105

CHAPTER 4: DIET RECIPES FOR PCOS 109

4.1 Breakfast 115

4.2 Lunch 127

4.3 Dinner 142

4.4 Sweets 165

4.5 Snacks and Smoothies 179

CONCLUSION 192

INTRODUCTION

PCOS IN A NUTSHELL

Polycystic ovary syndrome is a widespread hormonal disorder in reproductive women. PCOS women may have unusual or prolonged menstrual periods or elevated levels of the male hormone (androgen). The ovaries can produce multiple small fluid (follicles) collections and not release eggs regularly.

The unknown is the precise cause of PCOS. Early diagnosis and treatment, together with weight loss, may reduce the risk of long-term complications such as heart disease and diabetes type 2. Polycystic ovary syndrome (PCOS) affects the hormone level of a woman. Women with PCOS generate male hormones that are higher than average. This disparity in the hormone allows you to miss menstrual periods to get pregnant.

PCOS also induces facial and body hair development and baldness. It leads to long-term health problems, such as diabetes and cardiac disease.

Diabetes and birth control pills can help correct hormone imbalance and boost symptoms. PCOS is a hormone problem that affects women (age 15 to 44) during their childhood. In this age group, 2.2-26.7% of women are PCOS. Many women don't know PCOS, but many people have PCOS.

PCOS affects the ovaries of women, the reproductive organs containing estrogen and progesterone – hormones regulating the menstrual cycle. The ovaries also include a small number of male androgen hormones. The ovaries produce eggs for sperm fertilization. Each month, the release of an egg is called ovulation.

The FSH hormone and the luteinizing hormone (LH) ovulation regulate. FSH drives the ovary into a follicle — a sac holding an egg — and then the LH activates the ovary into a ripe egg.

PCOS is a "syndrome," or collection of ovarian and reproductive symptoms. The three main features are ovarian cysts with high levels of abnormal or missed male hormones. In the PCOS, a large number of small, fluid-filled bags develop inside the ovaries. The word polycystic means "multiple cysts." These sacs are follicles with an immature egg. The eggs never mature enough to induce ovulation.

Ovulation deficiency affects estrogen, progesterone, FSH, and LH levels. The levels of estrogen and progesterone are less than usual, while the androgen is higher than average. Extra male hormones interrupt the menstrual cycle, causing women with PCOS to have fewer cycles than usual.

It's not a new problem for PCOS. In 1721, doctors didn't know exactly what causes PCOS; the Italian physicist Antonio Vallisneri first identified its symptoms. They conclude that high levels of male hormones prevent ovaries from producing hormones and eggs. Gens, resistance to insulin, and inflammation have all been related to excess development of androgen. Up to 70% of women diagnosed with PCOS have insulin resistance, so their cells cannot properly use insulin. If cells cannot efficiently use insulin, the body's demand for insulin increases. The pancreas makes more insulin to make up for it. Additional insulin activates ovaries to produce more male hormones.

The primary cause of insulin resistance is obesity. Obesity and resistance to insulin can raise the risk of type 2 diabetes Women with PCOS also experience elevated rates of inflammation in the body.

Overweight can also cause inflammation. Studies have related excess inflammation to higher levels of androgen. Some women begin to see symptoms around the first mark. Others only discover PCOS after losing a lot of weight or after having trouble getting pregnant.

The most common signs of PCOS are irregular periods. A lack of ovulation prevents the lining of the uterus from falling every month. Some women are less than eight times a year with PCOS.

- Slow bleeding. The uterine lining is thicker, so the times you get can be lighter than average.
- Hair growth. Over 70 percent of the women with this condition develop hair, including on their back, belly, and chest on their face and body. Hirsutism is known as excess hair growth.
- The gain in weight. Up to 80% of PCOS females are overweight or obese.
- Baldness. Hair becomes thinner on the scalp and falls off.
- Skin darkening. Dark skin patches can develop like on the back, in the groin, and under the breasts in the body.
- Headaches. Changes in hormones can cause problems in some women.

Higher than normal levels of androgen will affect your fertility and other health aspects.

Infertility you have to ovulate to get pregnant. Women that do not routinely ovulate do not eat as many eggs to be fertilized. One of the most common causes of women's infertility is PCOS. Up to 80% of women with PCOS are overweight or obese. Metabolic syndrome. The risk of high blood sugar, high blood pressure, and low cholesterol ("good") HDL and high cholesterol LDL ("bad") also rises with PCOS. These causes are known as metabolic syndrome together, which raises the risk of heart disease, diabetes, and stroke.

This condition causes many night respiration delays that interrupt sleep, known as Sleep apnea. Sleep apnea is more common in overweight women — especially in women with PCOS. In obese women with PCOS, the incidence of sleep apnea is five to ten times higher than in those without PCOS. Endometrial cancer uterine lining sheds during ovulation. The lining will build up if you don't ovulate every month. A thickened uterine lining will increase your cancer risk. Depression Hormone changes and signs such as unwanted hair growth may affect your emotions. Depression Many with PCOS usually starts with lifestyle changes such as weight loss, diet, and exercise with PCOS depression and anxiety treatment. Losing only 5-10% of your weight will help to control your menstrual cycle and boost PCOS symptoms. Loss of weight can also raise cholesterol, reduce insulin, and lower the risk of heart disease and diabetes. Some foods, however, may have advantages over others. Studies comparing PCOS diets have shown that low-carbon diets are useful for both weight loss and decreased insulin levels. The low glycemic (low-GI) food that uses fruit, vegetables, and whole grains to get the most carbohydrates helps to regulate the menstrual cycle better than a regular diet of weight loss.

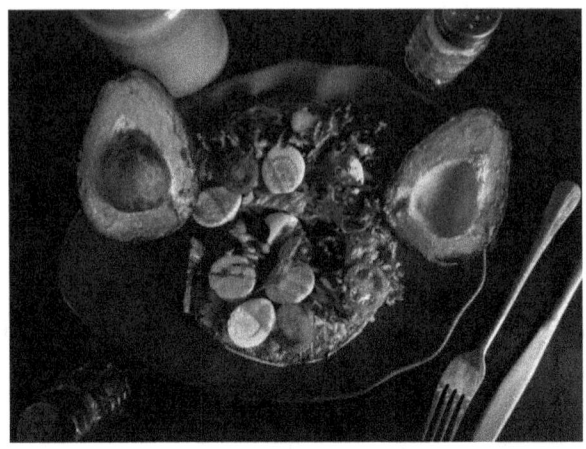

A few studies found that 30 minutes of moderate-intensity exercise would help women lose weight with PCOS, at least three days a week. The low pressure also increases ovulation and insulin levels with activity. Use, in combination with a healthy diet, is even more beneficial. Diet plus exercise will reduce the risk of diabetes and heart disease. There are some indications that acupuncture can help boost PCOS, but further research is required.

CHAPTER 1: DIAGNOSING AND UNDERSTANDING PCOS

There is no standard procedure to detect PCOS. The doctor will also continue thinking about personal history, including the menstrual cycle and weight shifts. Environmental monitoring may include looking for signs of premature hair growth, insulin resistance, and acne.

There is an option for a vaginal test. The doctor must physically and manually check the genital organs for masses, growths, or other anomalies.

Medical checks, yes. Blood can be tested to determine hormone levels. This examination can remove potential causes of menstrual irregularities or androgen overload that resemble PCOS. The patient may have additional blood tests to assess glucose absorption and low cholesterol and triglyceride levels.

Another option is an ultrasound. The doctor will test the size of your ovaries and the consistency of the lining of your uterus. A wand-like tool (transducer) is put in the vagina (transvaginal ultrasound). The transducer emits sound waves that are converted into images on a computer screen.

When you have a diagnosis of PCOS, further complications testing can be prescribed by the doctor. Other measures can include regular blood pressure testing, glucose tolerances, and cholesterol and triglyceride rates—monitoring for stress and anxiety.

Lifestyle improvements: The doctor can prescribe weight loss by a low-calorie diet paired with regular exercise. Just a small reduction in your weight — for example, a loss of 5% of your body weight — may improve your health. Losing weight can also improve the potency of PCOS drugs prescribed by the doctor, which can assist with infertility.

Medications: The doctor may recommend a combination of birth control pills to manage the menstrual cycle. Medicines containing estrogen and progestin reduce the production of androgen and control the production of testosterone. Regulation of your hormones will reduce the risk of endometrial cancer and correct excessive bleeding, premature hair growth, and acne. You may use a skin patch or a vaginal ring that includes a mixture of estrogen and progestin instead of tablets.

Therapy of progestin. Getting progestin 10 to 14 days every one or two months monitors your period and prevents you from endometrial cancer. Progestin therapy will not raise androgen levels and does not prevent abortion. A progestin-only maniple or progestin-containing intrauterine system is a safer option if you do choose to avoid abortion.

1.1 Effects of Diet on PCOS

What to eat if you have PCOS Polycystic Ovarian Syndrome is a disorder that triggers hormonal imbalances and metabolic issues.

Polycystic ovarian syndrome (PCOS) is a common health condition encountered by one in ten women of childbearing age. PCOS can also contribute to other severe health issues, such as diabetes, respiratory disorders, insomnia, and an elevated chance of endometrial cancer.

Some work has shown that diet can help to reduce the effects of PCOS.

How does the diet affect PCOS?

People with PCOS can benefit from a diet that includes high-fiber foods.

Weight control and insulin development and tolerance are two of the main ways that diet impacts PCOS.

Nevertheless, insulin plays a significant role in PCOS, and controlling insulin levels in PCOS is one of the first steps patients can do to treat the disease.

A lot of people with PCOS have insulin resistance. More than 50% of people with PCOS experience diabetes or prediabetes before the age of 40. Diabetes is linked explicitly to the way the body produces insulin.

A diet that satisfies the food needs of a person maintains a stable weight and encourages proper insulin levels can make people with PCOS feel better.

Foods to eat

The study has shown that what people consume has a significant impact on PCOS. That said, there is no regular PCOS diet.

However, there is a consensus as to which foods are helpful and tend to help people control their illness and which foods to prevent.

- Low Glycemic Index (GI) Diet: The body slowly digests low GI foods to ensure that they do not cause the amount of insulin to rise as much or as rapidly as other foods, such as specific carbon dioxide. Low-GI products include whole grains, legumes, almonds, pears, baits, starchy foods, and other low-carbohydrates unprocessed foods.

- Anti-inflammatory diet, which can reduce inflammatory symptoms such as weakness, including vegetables, Fatty fish, leafy greens, and extra virgin olive oil.

- DASH diet: Physicians also prescribe Medical Strategies to Avoid Hypertension (Dot) diets to reduce the risk or effect of heart failure. This can also help to relieve the impact of PCOS. The diet of DASH is abundant in fish, meat, fruit, whole grain vegetables, and low-fat dairy products. Foods that are rich in saturated fat and sugar are avoided by diet. A 2015 report showed that obese women who followed a specially formulated DASH diet for eight weeks had a decrease in insulin tolerance and belly fat relative to those who did not follow the same menu.

Proper PCOS diet can also contain the following ingredients:

- raw, unprocessed ingredients
    - fatty fish like salmon, tuna, sardines, and mackerel
    - kale, spinach and another fatty, leafy grasses
    - dark green fruits such as red raisins, blueberry, blackberry, and cerise
    - broccoli and cauliflower

- dried beans, lentils, and other vegetables
- healthy fats, succulents
- Individuals lose more weight on a diet that favors monounsaturated fats rather than saturated fats. An example of this kind of food is the anti-inflammatory diet, which allows people to consume vegetable fats, such as olive oils and other vegetable oils.
- People who followed a low-carbohydrate or low-GI diet saw improved insulin metabolism and lower levels of cholesterol. People with PCOS who adopted a low-GI diet have indicated a more exceptional quality of life and more frequent periods.
- Studies have shown that weight loss benefits people with PCOS, regardless of the particular form of diet they adopt.

Foods to avoid

Sharing with People on a PCOS diet should avoid sugary beverages.

Those on the PCOS diet should eliminate food that is commonly perceived as unhealthful.

- Processed carbs, such as mass-produced pastries and white bread.

- New food, such as fast meals.
- Sugary beverages, such as energy drinks and sodas.
- Processed foods, such as hot dogs, sausages, and burgers for lunch.
- Strong fat, like margarine, shortening, and lard.
- Needless fried meat, such as steaks, hamburgers, and bacon.

Lifestyle changes will also help people with PCOS control their disease. Evidence has demonstrated that mixing a PCOS diet with physical exercise will contribute to the following benefits:

- weight reduction
- increased insulin absorption
- more frequent cycles
- decreased rates of male hormones and male model hair development
- Lower levels of cholesterol. Researchers have also shown that lifestyle approaches may help women achieve weight control goals that, in effect.

These activities include:

- goal-setting

- peer support networks
- self-monitoring strategies
- psychological wellbeing treatment

Mitigating tension by self-care habits, such as having a night of adequate sleep, preventing over-commitment, and finding time to relax, will also help a person handle PCOS. Common PCOS symptoms include:

- acne
- excess hair growth
- weight gain, particularly around the abdomen
- oily skin
- erratic cycles
- pain in the pelvic region
- trouble getting pregnant

Some people who have such symptoms do not find them severe enough to speak to a doctor. Most people don't receive professional attention because they have a rough time conceiving. Anyone who has these symptoms will address their issues with the doctor: The quicker a treatment plan can be completed, the quicker one can feel better.

While PCOS is not healed at this time, people can their symptoms and enhance their quality of life by taking a healthy diet and being physically active.

A person's control of PCOS will help to reach and maintain a healthy weight and consume healthy fats, lean proteins, and a reasonable amount of low-GI carbohydrate.

1.2 Foods to Consume

Polycystic Ovarian Syndrome (PCOS) is a hormonal syndrome that affects 1 in 10 people but is frequently misdiagnosed or confused, causing other people to suffer in silence. Whether you have been infected with PCOS or have been suffering from the disorder for many years, a variety of interventions can help alleviate and ease the symptoms, including bio identical hormone replacement treatment and diet. Here are some of the things to be consumed with PCOS and others to avoid!

Know, before you change your diet or lifestyle to treat the effects of PCOS, it is often wise to contact a hormone expert for treatment and advice. For hormonal disorders, there is often rarely a 'one size fits all' approach, so careful monitoring will help decide which diet is better suited to the particular hormone levels.

Although diet cannot be a complete solution, tests have demonstrated that if a patient with PCOS loses weight, their symptoms will change. Diet and diet play a significant role in weight control, and so paying attention to what you eat and adjusting it accordingly can help with the symptoms of PCOS. Many people with this particular condition find that low-carb, high-protein diet is very successful for weight loss with PCOS.

But, it isn't just about weight, as the foods you consume will affect your hormone output directly, and so eating those foods will help to reduce your symptoms at hormone level. When you're thinking about what foods to eat with PCOS, it's essential to consider every aspect of your diet from breakfast to dinner, to ensure you're eating a balanced diet and keeping a lot of variety that can make healthy eating a lot easier to stick to.

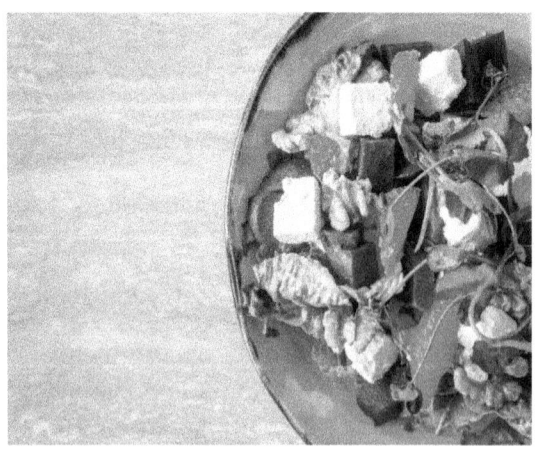

If you have been diagnosed with PCOS, pay attention to adding these foods to your diet!

No matter what diet you start, green leafy vegetation is the right call. They are nutrient-rich and calorie-low and are suitable for both weight loss and food consumption. Most notably, however, green leafy plants, such as kale or spinach, contain high concentrations of vitamin B for those with PCOS. Incredibly, more than 80% of people with PCOS are vitamin B deficient! This particular vitamin is linked to many symptoms of PCOS, including:

- Insulin Resistance
- Irregular Periods
- Hirsutism (excess hair growth)
- Obesity
- Difficulty Designing

Healthy Grass-Fed Meat

This is particularly true for patients with PCOS who may find weight loss more difficult due to hormonal imbalances.

Eating grass-fed, organic beef is just as important as keeping an eye on the food's fat content. Non-organic meat usually consists of higher levels of hormones given to livestock, which can have a direct impact on human hormone levels. Fresh beef, on the other hand, typically has far lower levels of animal hormones, making it easier to consume if you have a hormonal imbalance.

Avocadoes

There are many healthier fats you can include in your diet, from avocados to fatty fish, which are especially suitable for eating with PCOS. Good fats are a source of essential fatty acids that are core components of cell wall maintenance. Not just that, but they are the secret to maintaining the correct balancing of your hormones, as well as regulating your weight.

Fertility is a significant problem for women who undergo PCOS and pregnancy and fatty acids play an essential part in all of these. Omega 3, a fatty acid that can be contained in foods such as seafood or linseed, helps

- Control hormones
- Decrease the body's exposure to prolactin, a hormone that may inhibit ovulation
- Improve blood flow to the uterus
- Raise egg white cervical mucus that lets sperm enter the egg

- Help manage the menstrual period, and this may increase the likelihood of having pros.

They help, for example, to support a healthy circulatory and nervous system!

Berries, seeds, green tea (anything rich in antioxidants!)

Well, so that might be a broad category, so you will find a list of the top ten healthy antioxidant foods here. These include Gobi Berries, blueberries, dark chocolate, and pecans, all of which contain high amounts of antioxidants. Although these foods are all essential for a balanced diet, in any case, they have even greater importance if you have PCOS.

People with PCOS have been found to have a higher degree of oxidative stress, which can then be combated by consuming more elevated amounts of antioxidants in our food. When selecting these products, it is essential to look at them about their glycemic index (GI) because certain fruits that cause a spike in blood sugar levels that may have consequences for PCOS-related diabetes.

Wholegrain

Women who suffer from PCOS are four times more likely to develop type 2 diabetes, and whole grains consist of high levels of fiber, which can help manage insulin levels.

High fiber foods, such as peas, beans, almonds, dried fruit, or wholegrain rice, are slow-release carbohydrates. This means that they release insulin to the blood at a steady, more reasonable rate and are thus less likely to induce increases of blood sugar associated with type 2 diabetes.

1.3 Foods to Limit or Avoid

These are foods that can be avoided or reduced if you have been diagnosed with PCOS. Glycemic Index (GI) that is directly related to insulin production and diabetes. As has already been mentioned, women with PCOS are much more likely to develop diabetes, and therefore it is essential to avoid high GI foods that are likely to lead to a spike in your blood sugars. It includes fried foods such as pies, cookies, and ready meals, but also contains carbs such as white potatoes, white bread, and white rice.

Milk products

You need to understand the role of Insulin Growth Factor 1 (IGF-1) to know why you should avoid PCOS milk. The post provides an excellent summary, just to simplify IGF-1 mimics the function and position of insulin in the body, so it has been found that women with PCOS have far higher rates of IGF-1 than most individuals. The IGF-1 present in cow's milk products has the same function as human IFG-1 and thus raises these amounts in the body.

Unhealthy Fats

We've already established that 'healthy fats' can play a decisive role in PCOS management, and the opposite is exact for 'bad fats.' Foods that have saturated or hydrogenated fats include dairy products such as cream or cheese and fatty red meat, as well as processed or fried foods. Such unhealthy fats may increase the development of estrogen, which may exacerbate your symptoms of PCOS, which may contribute to weight gain, which may also worsen your symptoms.

Soy products

Soy products have been shown to increase estrogen levels, which is excellent for anyone with low estrogen levels but can be detrimental to those with PCOS or other dominant estrogen conditions. Although there is still some controversy over the effect of soybean on estrogen levels, it is worth considering taking out soybean products if you suffer from PCOS.

Gluten

This is because gluten can lead to inflammation that can lead to insulin resistance and increase your risk of developing diabetes. Those with higher levels of inflammation have also been shown to have excess production of androgen, which can contribute to weight gain and irregular menstruation, both of which are common symptoms of PCOS.

What to do next

"What's next?" You have all this knowledge about what to eat with PCOS, so what are you going to do with it? The most important thing you have to do before anything else is speaking to your doctor about your options. Many women living with PCOS will be recommended to change their diet. Although this information is helpful, more therapies should be provided to facilitate these changes. For example, bio-identical hormone replacement therapy (BHRT) can be an ideal choice for treating or even removing PCOS symptoms. Bio-identical hormones, as their name suggests, are structurally identical to your hormones and are derived from plants. After a proper diagnosis and analysis of your hormone test findings, the BHRT specialist will recommend the exact hormone levels required to stabilize your endocrine system better.

At the very least, in addition to changing your diet, it is also essential to seek professional recommendations and consider all your choices from a dietary and medical viewpoint.

1.4 Other Lifestyle Changes To Consider

Diet and lifestyle are the primary approaches to treatment for women with PCOS. Here are the five main components of a balanced PCOS lifestyle.

You know that PCOS requires a balanced diet, but exactly what does that mean? Women with PCOS have higher inflammatory rates that trigger hormone imbalances (low testosterone rates, hormone luteinization, and insulin).

An inflammation-focused diet works well for PCOS women. The anti-inflammatory diet includes many fruits and vegetables, small quantities of fiber-free, unprepared low-GI grains (oats, quinoa), and omega-3-rich foods such as fish (salmon, tuna, trout), almonds, bohemians, and avocados.

One significant feature of a healthy PCOS diet is the standardized distribution of carbohydrate calories during the day, rather than at once. This helps in blood sugar levels regulation and increased insulin spikes. Eat around one-fourth of your plate, moderate quantities of carbohydrate per meal, and snack for nutrition. Eat moderate amounts of sugar per meal and snack, about one-quarter of your plate, for balance.

Regularly Diet exercise alone is not enough to manage PCOS properly. Since they have higher levels of testosterone, people with PCOS appear to build muscle more quickly than those without the disorder. More muscle mass increases the metabolic rate, so you burn calories more efficiently, and it helps you better use glucose, which means less insulin needs to be secreted. Aim to do at least two days of weight lifting per week to develop and retain muscle mass. Adding extra exercise to your day by taking the stairs instead of the elevator, moving the car away from the entrance, or taking quick walks at lunch or breaks will make a difference to your wellbeing and help you generate less insulin. Some people find it useful to use fitness trackers to step up every day and even interact with peers or friends.

Getting a lot of sleep or lack of sleep can have a significant impact on the health of women with PCOS. Lack of Sleep is associated with decreased insulin resistance and weight loss problems. Insufficient sleep has also been linked with a higher intake of processed food.

People with PCOS have been found to have higher levels of obstructive sleep apnea (OSA), a disorder that induces a loss in breathing throughout sleep. Although extra weight can be an OSA cause, elevated testosterone levels that affect sleep receptors in the brain are also a concern. If you have been advised to snore if you don't get enough sleep or have excessive exhaustion during the day, recommend having a sleep analysis done to check for OSA. Treatment typically requires using a CPAP machine, which will result in you getting more stamina and better time dropping weight.

Having a handle on tension is part of everyone's day. Constant prolonged stress, if not managed, can cause significant health problems, such as high blood pressure, and can lead to an increase in cortisol and insulin levels that contribute to weight gain.

If you find like you can't hang on to your pressures, try a pressure control plan focused on mindfulness that can help you cope with tension more efficiently. Daily exercise, meditation, or yoga is practices that can reduce the levels of cortisol and insulin in women with PCOS.

Manage PCOS weight women will have more trouble losing weight with PCOS. After all, insulin is an appetite stimulant that facilitates fat accumulation, and many women with conditions have quickly increased their pressure.

The critical elements of a healthy PCOS lifestyle discussed here help to lose weight. Fad diets that promote drastic loss of weight only add to the yo-yo diet process. Seek to contact a certified dietitian who is trained in PCOS to regulate your pressure.

1.5 Research Findings Of nutritional Diet Plan for PCOS

Diet and rehabilitation are critical aspects of the treatment of PCOS (Polycystic Ovarian Syndrome). This is because young ladies with PCOS also have higher insulin (hormone) in their blood and often find it hard to keep their body weight safely. Understanding the best kinds of food to consume and the best types of food to consume will change the way you look and can help you lose weight? Eating well, being active, and keeping a good weight (or only dropping a slight amount of weight if you are overweight) will reduce the effects of PCOS.

How do you know about lepton and carbohydrates?

After you have eaten, the amount of insulin in your blood is rising. It's the most important thing when you eat or drink something that includes carbohydrates. Carbohydrates are present in grains (such as flour, pasta, rice, and cereal), most snack foods (such as popcorn, cookies, and candy), sugary beverages such as soda and milk, and fruit and vegetables.

Also, if you eat two foods containing the same amount of glucose, they can have a significant impact on your insulin level. This shift is more related to the number of carbohydrates produced by the food. Carbohydrate foods containing antioxidants, such as whole wheat, fruit, and vegetables, are typically the safest things to consume while you're working to keep the insulin levels down. Carbohydrate foods that are sugary or processed (such as soda, water, white bread, and white rice) can increase insulin levels. Meals and drinks like this are often not very whole (which means that you can feel thirsty shortly after you eat them). Seek to pick high-fiber, low-sugar starch meals most of the time.

You don't have to leave the way to buy different products. The diet would be a combination of vegetables, nuts, whole grains, vegetable proteins, maize, and healthy fats, as with any balanced eating program. Most foods are a healthy diet for PCOS, but you should read food labels to make better choices. Look for high-fiber grains like brown rice, whole-wheat, and whole-wheat bread instead of fiber-thin grains like white rice, pasta, or white bread.

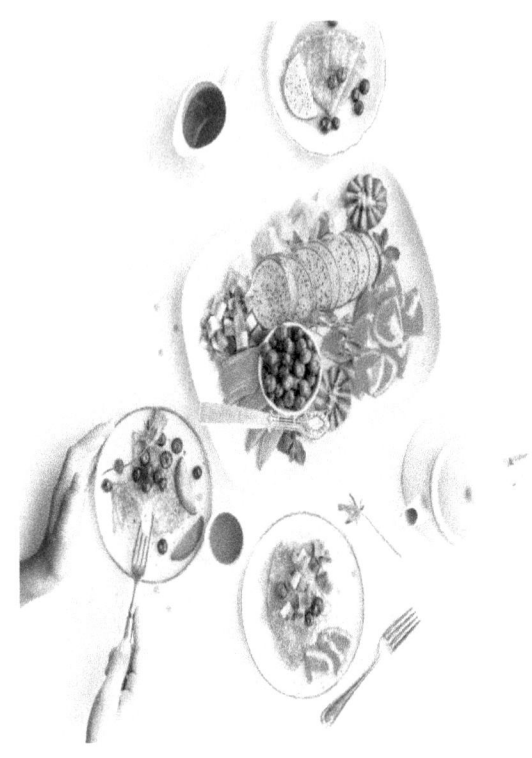

Don't be fooled by counseling without fat. They generally have a lot of sugar added to them. Additionally, certain sugar-free foods (such as baked goods) are made from processed grains such as white flour, which can raise the insulin levels in the same manner as sugar does. Many sugar-free diets are free of sugars. These foods, sweetened with artificial sweetener, maybe a good alternative if your stomach is not upset. There are currently no scientific data suggesting that moderate amounts of artificial sweetener are harmful to our health. These foods and beverages are refined, however. Aim to adhere to the most objective, entire type of each meal (i.e., the lemon cut in water instead of lemonade).

- Sweetened Milk, dried fruit in thick syrup or sweetened apple sauce

- Starchy crops such as carrots, corn, and peas

- Refined foods made with white flour such as white bread and spaghetti, bagels or white rice Foods such as Lucky Charms ®, Fruit Loops ® or Frosted Flakes ® and other sweetened grains such as chocolate bars (Nutrigrain Bars ®), snack pastry (Pop Tar Bars ®) (Search for 5 grams of fiber cereals per serving or sprinkle 1/2 cup bran with low fiber maize to improve fiber)

- milk or lard, flavored with fruit if desired, non-sweetened ice-creams

- High fiber baked goods made of wheat flour and oat

- Cracks and treats like Trip ®, Wasa ® or popcorn carbs (carbohydrates).

Many other essential nutrients, such as vitamins and minerals, come from starchy foods, but having no carbohydrates is not a smart idea. Since high-fiber-carbohydrate carbohydrates are rich in nutrients and make you stay full longer than low-fiber carbohydrate sugars, it is better to use high-fiber carbs as much as possible.

Nutrition foods such as beans, hummus, almonds, peanut butter, tofu, bacon, fish, chicken, beef and vegetarian beef alternatives, and fats such as olive oil, almonds, and avocado are essential aspects of the PCOS-friendly diet program. Combining foods containing protein or fat with carbohydrates can help to reduce the absorption of carbohydrates and keep insulin small. For starters, instead of plain rice, have a little bean rice and a little avocado.

Bear in mind that some fats are a lot safer than others. Good fats can be found in olive oil, canola oil, almonds, avocados, and fish. Choose balanced fats and proteins instead of butter, margarine, mayonnaise, full-bodied cheese, fluffy sauces or dressings, and red meat. The diets of the high protein (such as the Atkins diet) for teens are not an excellent diet because they are low in essential nutrients such as fiber, B vitamins, and vitamin C. It should also be kept in mind that even though you restrict your carbohydrate intake, excessive fat or protein will lead to a gain in weight. You will look for a food that has a combination of protein, balanced carbohydrates, and fat.

The glycemic index is a terminology used to describe the effects of food on blood sugar. The higher the ingested blood sugar, the higher the glycemic index. The glycemic index of high fiber carbs is lower than that for sugar or refined carbs. Combining carbohydrate food with another food will reduce the glycemic index by allowing the body to digest glucose more slowly. E.g., if you eat a piece of candy right after a meal, it won't raise your blood sugar as much as it wills if you ate the candy on your own between meals.

Vegetables such as asparagus, broccoli, cabbage, cauliflower, celery, cucumber, green beans, lettuce, tomatoes and zucchini, and fruit such as bananas, berries, grapes, strawberries, peaches, and plums provide a low glycemic level. Some sugar or starch fruit and vegetable products have a higher degree of glycaemia (like canned berries, tropical fruit, beans, cold cuts, squash, peas).

There is no existing clinical evidence to endorse reducing or restricting different food classes or food types to enhance the effects of PCOS. Using the nutritional recommendations given here, in addition to exercise, there are safe ways to control weight and reduce symptoms.

Besides what you consume, how much you consume also influences the amount of insulin. For starters, if you have 3 cups of pasta, your insulin will increase much more than if you have one pasta bowl. This means that it's generally more comfortable to have a few small meals and snacks throughout the day than to have a few huge meals. Having more regular smaller meals and snacks will keep the insulin rates lower all day.

The label with nutritional facts describes what nutrients (food components the body requires to develop and remain healthy) and how many of them are present in a portion of a meal. This is located on the exterior of most food packets, but not on most fresh foods (such as fruit and vegetables or meats). The Nutrition Facts label may help you make choices about the food you eat.

The mark shall include any or more of the following nutrients:

- Serving Size: Serving Size represents one serving of the food. All other nutrient values on the label are based on this amount.

- Tub Servings: This figure is how many servings you would receive from a single box. Few packages have one meal, but most of them have more than one serving per box.

- •Calories (total): Calories are an energy unit that is extracted from carbohydrates, proteins, and fat.

Calories give us the strength and energy we need to think.

- Fat calories: This is the number of calories that come from fat. It's not the percentage of fat in the food.

- Percent Daily Weight: Which is the amount of the average daily weight of the nutrient that you get with one serving? Food containing more than 20% of the Daily Value of a Nutrient is an outstanding source; but, the lower the amount, the better for other nutrients such as sugar, sodium, and cholesterol.

- Total fat: fat is essential to our bodies. There are four kinds of fat. Monounsaturated and polyunsaturated fats are the kind of fat that is healthy for the heart.

- Tran's fat: Trans-fat is not healthy for your heart and should be avoided.

- Cholesterol: Cholesterol is a substance found only in animal products. Overeating cholesterol is not suitable for your heart.

- Sodium: Sodium is the amount of salt contained in the consumption of food. Individuals with elevated blood pressure are frequently advised to take a low sodium diet.

- Absolute Carbohydrate: Carbohydrates give energy to your brain and muscles. Some forms of carbohydrates are also labeled.

- Dietary Fiber: improves digestion and leaves you fresh between meals.

- Sugars: are essential for instant energy, but consuming too much added sugar could be unhealthful. The Nutrition Facts label will soon list naturally occurring sugar (such as the lactose in milk) separately from artificial sugar (such as cocoa in chocolate milk).

- Protein: this element is used to create muscles and combat infections.

- Vitamins and Minerals (A, C, Calcium, and Iron): This is the proportion (percent) of the daily amount of vitamin A, vitamin C, calcium, and iron that you get from the serving of this drink. Many vitamins and minerals can also be included in this portion.

Many ingredients, such as polyunsaturated or monounsaturated fat and other vitamins and minerals, can also be listed on the Nutrition Facts label because the organization that manufactures the product requires them.

The first thing you can look at is the scale of the serving. The sum of each nutrient on the package is what is contained in one serving of the product, not in the entire bottle. If you don't know what the size of a meal is, you won't see the sum of every nutrient you receive. For starters, there are three servings in a large bag of microwave popcorn. It's all right to take more than one portion at a time, so it's good to remember that if you consume the entire package, you'll get three times what's on the bottle. Section control is an integral aspect of balanced PCOS feeding, so bear in mind the size of the section.

Given this, you don't need to keep track of any food you consume. Only take a look at the Nutrition Facts label once in a while to help you make healthier decisions and select foods that can give the body the nutrients it needs. For example, if you don't drink a lot of milk, you can read the Nutrition Facts label to help you identify specific foods and beverages that are rich in calcium. You can also use the Nutrition Facts sticker to compare two different meals. For example, if you choose between two different types of bread, reading the Nutrition Facts labels will help you make a better decision. Consider selecting the food that has the highest fiber content.

A 2000-calorie diet may be perfect for you, but many teens require more than 2,000 calories as they grow tall, develop bones, build muscles, and remain healthy, and others may need a little less. The 2000-calorie diet is just an approximation that is used to measure the percent (percent) Caloric Amount on the Nutrition Facts tab.

It's also essential for girls to treat PCOS because treat decreases insulin levels, can help with weight control, is suitable for cardiovascular health, and can help to change their mood. Exercise can be particularly helpful in lowering insulin right after a meal. And, if possible, go for a stroll or find a fun way to move your body after you've had a meal. Any increase in exercise helps to find the activity, sport, or use you enjoy. If you're not doing a lot of training right now, start slowly and focus on your fitness target. If you work out just once in a while, try to exercise more frequently. Work to increase your physical activity to at least five days a week for 60 minutes a day.

1.6 What You Should Know About PCOS and Fertility

A polycystic ovarian syndrome is a condition diagnosed with a deficiency of female sex hormones by doctors. The disparity can contribute to several symptoms and can affect the fertility of an individual.

Every month, tiny, fluid-filled cysts known as follicles grow on the surface of the ovaries in women of childbearing age. Female sex hormones, including estrogen, allow one of the follicles to release a mature egg. Then the ovary releases the nucleus and it bursts free of the follicle.

There is a difference between female sex hormones of people with polycystic ovarian syndrome or PCOS. The imbalance will prevent the production and release of mature eggs. No ovulation or pregnancy may occur without a mature egg.

Hormone deficiency can also include an excessive rise in testosterone, which is predominantly a male sex hormone. Women do contain testosterone, but it is typically small in number.

The Office for Women's Health (OWH) of the United States reports that PCOS affects 5-10 percent of women aged 15-44 years. PCOS is described as a "normal and treatable cause of infertility." Sharing causes of PCOS may contribute to changes in facial hair and skin health. Genetic influences can have a role to play.

Experts may not know exactly what causes PCOS, but they can include genetic factors. When a woman's mother or sister has a disease, she has a better risk of having it than most.

In addition to the genetic relation, excess insulin in the body also raises a woman's risk of developing PCOS. Insulin is emitted from the pancreas and used by the organism to turn sugar into food energy.

People with PCOS also have resistance to insulin. Insulin tolerance means that the body is unable to reduce blood sugar levels correctly. Blood sugar levels can get too high, which causes further insulin production.

Too much insulin also increases the development of testosterone, which contributes to some effects of PCOS.

Signs

Signs can appear at any age or period in a person's reproductive years. Symptoms can also alter over time.

Many of the more prominent effects with PCOS include:

- excessive hair development on the neck, back or chest
- acne or darkening of the skin
- weight gain
- thinning of the hair on the head

- miscarriage
- prolonged cycles
- ovarian cysts
- insomnia
- Elevated skin marks not all with PCOS may experience the same indications or effects.

Effects on PCOS fertility can influence a person's productivity in several ways

Ovulation complications are typically the primary cause of infertility in people with PCOS. Ovulation may not occur due to increased production of testosterone or because ovarian follicles do not mature.

Even if ovulation occurs, a hormone imbalance can prevent the lining of the uterus from forming correctly so that the mature egg can be implanted.

Ovulation and menstruation can be abnormal due to imbalanced hormones. Unpredictable menstrual periods will also make it impossible to get pregnant.

Other complications often, infertility are one of the main difficulties of PCOS, but not the only one.

Women with PCOS do tend to have a higher chance than those of

- elevated cholesterol rates
- high blood pressure
- cardiac failure
- diabetes
- weight gain
- sleep apnea
- depression and anxiety
- weak self-confidence
- endometrial cancer

According to the OWH, approximately half of the people with PCOS experience either prediabetes or diabetes by age 40.

Everyone concerned about being unable to get pregnant or symptoms indicating that PCOS should see a doctor. Even if a woman is unable to become pregnant, early PCOS diagnosis will help to avoid complications.

There are several alternative causes of infertility, but PCOS diagnosis may improve treatment and conceivability.

When a woman is pregnant, it is, therefore, essential to know when PCOS is involved, as tests have indicated a higher risk of pregnancy problems with PCOS.

These risks can include

- gestational diabetes
- early birth
- Elevated blood pressure during breastfeeding.

There is no clinical test to detect PCOS. A doctor makes a decision based on a variety of variables.

Tests can include

- Physical exam
- Psychiatric history
- Blood checks for hormone levels
- Blood tests for glucose level
- Mir scan Therapy

There is currently no cure for PCOS. Treatment may, however, increase the chances of conception for those who wish to become pregnant. It will also help patients control their symptoms.

Symptoms vary between people, and diagnosis is not necessarily the same. Options may depend on whether or not a person chooses to become pregnant.

Treatment of symptoms of PCOs can include:

- Birth control pills to help fix hormone imbalances.
- Insulin-sensitizing medications to enhance the body's use of insulin and hence thus the production of testosterone.
- Medication to regulate blood sugar levels in the event of diabetes.
- Sleep and balanced food to help improve physical wellbeing and regulate weight.

Maintaining a proper weight will help to reduce insulin and testosterone levels and boost symptoms.

Fertility treatment for PCOS When a woman wants to become pregnant, a doctor can recommend medications to control menstrual cycles and promote ovulation. Surgery can be an alternative if the drugs do not boost fertility.

Laparoscopic ovary drilling is a surgical choice. In this operation, the surgeon makes minor holes in the abdomen and attaches an electrical current needle.

They use electrical current to remove a small amount of tissue that contains ovarian testosterone. Decreased levels of testosterone can require frequent ovulation to occur.

Weight management

For people who are overweight, weight loss will better improve hormone development and increase the likelihood of ovulation and pregnancy.

According to the OWH, only a 10% weight loss can enable an individual with excess weight and fertility problems to regain their regular ovulation.

People of low weight who have trouble conceiving will still want to visit a doctor, as that may be another potential factor for infertility.

Managing stress

Seeking safe ways to relieve depression will also improve fertility.

Long-term stress may affect hormones. For example, continuing pressure may increase cortisol in the body, which may contribute to an increase in insulin production. High insulin levels can contribute to imbalances in female sex hormones and infertility.

Stress reduction strategies include:

- having enough exercise
- juggling job and home life

- spending time with friends and family
- getting adequate sleep

Nutritional adjustments for specific individuals with PCOS, a low glycemic diet can boost symptoms and fertility.

A low glycemic diet means consuming fewer items that induce an increase in blood sugar.

Avoiding surges ensures that blood sugar levels are more stable, resulting in lower insulin levels and lower testosterone production.

Other factors influencing PCOS reproduction are just one of the several potential causes of female infertility. Any specific objectives include endometriosis: uterine tissue development outside the uterus can also contribute to infertility, mainly as it occurs in the fallopian tubes.

Structural problems: The issue with the construction of fallopian tubes or other parts of the reproduction system may make it difficult to become pregnant.

Fibroids: These uterine cancer tumors can cause fertility problems by preventing implantation.

However, several women with fertility problems — including PCOS — may become pregnant with medical support.

The first way to improve the risk of abortion is for a patient to see a doctor and have a correct diagnosis. They will continue therapy as early as possible by doing so.

CHAPTER 2: PCOS AND PHYSICAL FITNESS

There is no question about it: PCOS is correlated with being overweight. More than half of PCOS patients are obese. Recent research has also shown that if you are overweight, your chances of having PCOS are about five times higher than if you are healthy.

This chapter goes into detail on how to lose weight if you have PCOS and how to overcome some of the obstacles that come your way. If you have PCOS, you may need to oversee your weight, if you don't reduce it by a certain amount. You will find in this chapter how to maintain a low-GI diet (see Chapter 4), but tailor it to weight loss as well. This chapter also looks at dealing with hunger and cravings, which are particularly healthy if you live with PCOS.

Deciding how quickly to lose your dietitian or psychiatrist may have already offered you a minimum weight to meet or you may choose to set your minimum. The most practical and logical solutions to goal setting can be found in this section.

You will find your BMI by going to www.nhlbisupport.com/bmi and entering your height and weight in your BMI calculator.

If you would instead do the math yourself (have a calculator ready!), follow these three simple steps: 1. Measure the height in inches and subtract the number on its own.

E.g., if you are 5'6 "tall, that's 66 inches. Therefore, you subtract 66 × 66 = 4.356. 2. Quantify the weight in pounds and subtract by 703. E.g., if you are 160 pounds, you multiply 160 × 703 = 112.480. 3. Split the result in Phase 2 by addressing Phase 1. Use our running example, 112.480 = 4.356 = 25.8. That's BMI.

2.1 Shedding the Extra Load

You already do realize that if you have PCOS, it becomes more challenging to lose weight. Nobody understands precisely why, but there may be a combination of: usually, you get a lower metabolic rate to only melt the fat that much quicker.

Just be hungry and more vulnerable to food cravings such that raising the diet becomes more challenging for you.

The higher circulating insulin rates will make you more prone than consuming excess fuel as fat.

While losing weight is never straightforward, it may make the process simpler or at least less stressful following the recommendations outlined in the next pages.

Rule# 1: Gradual weight loss

The gradual weight loss is safer than fast weight loss because you have PCOS unless your doctor has informed you that weight loss is an immediate need. This is desirable to drop 1 or 2 pounds a week. The lack of weight will be done mainly though you are suffering from eating. Weight loss gradually is, therefore, less likely to be regained, so you are less inclined to drop weight, restore it, drop more, etc.

Rule # 2: Find the right food group

Rather than creating your menu and ensuring whether both amounts are following calorie counts (and therefore the rates of fat and Sucre are not out of balance), you may choose to try an "off the shelf" plan or see a dietitian receive advice. Search out a healthy diet schedule to see how many calories it contains.

Commercial weight reduction services, including weight tracking, may be beneficial, but remind them that you have PCOS and want to adopt a low GI system. Most services recognize this definition and will be able to provide some constructive guidance.

Web-based nutrition and blogs may be beneficial — some also offer low GI diets. You may have to pay to participate, but sometimes they are more comfortable than holding meetings in person. Many places provide a chat room for users. Again, diet guidance is reasonable and meets the recommendations contained in this book before entering the companion.

Few simple tips that might be considered:

- Avoid diets that report tremendous weight reductions within a short period.
- If a diet is scheduled for more than a month, about 1,500 calories a day is a sufficient consumption. If you have fewer than 15 pounds to lose for a shorter time, you will decrease to 1,300 calories. Don't get fewer than 1,200 calories.
- Avoid diets to eliminate other products or food classes. Stop diets that only support a limited number of items. Making sure the food is not a low-carbon food.
- Test that the meal schedule can also be tailored to a low-GI meal.

While you seem to have lost weight with specific treatments and medications, they are just partial remedies due to water depletion. When you drink regularly for a day or two, the pressure will go back because you haven't lost fat. You can also see claims that certain natural chemicals could make you lose weight, including caffeine and other stimulants. Green tea extracts Conjugated linoleic acid, a type of fat that is naturally present in the following techniques, make you lose weight but don't lose fat: body saunas or steam rooms.

Stimulants like caffeine are not generally accepted by anyone and can contribute to elevated blood pressure and other complications in safety.

Recording your weight and body fat in combination with your diet

You will instead compare the weight of the food to have a real understanding of cause and effect.

Weigh yourself only once a week, because weight can vary a lot every day. Try to do it with the same type of clothing or no clothes at the same time of day.

Consider investing in an amount that measures the fat percentage of your body. These scales are costlier than ordinary levels, but they give you a better picture of what happens while you lose weight. When you do follow a fitness regimen, you may notice that you lose more body fat than weight proportionally. This is because some of the body fat is not only burnt off; it is used to produce more muscle and loads more than fat. Moreover, if you work out, you could appear more toned and slender than a woman who doesn't work out.

To help your body notice and be content with a meal, take the time to enjoy thoroughly what you placed in your mouth. Seek to be mindful of any bite you take-you may start thinking that at the moment; you just don't want to consume the specific meal. You can even learn more when you feel complete and can set your knife down without anything needing to finish on your plate.

Enjoying the diet will make you consume fewer. Here are some tips on how to enjoy your food more: take an opportunity to have your meal.

Always sure that you consume food that is genuinely good and healthy. Don't place some old fast food in your mouth actively.

Just fill food or walk anywhere. Correctly set down at a table while you snack. Use a plate and utensils (even if you have a meal only).

Exception: It is recommended to communicate with your families and friends. (After all, you can't talk entirely through your mouth!) Eat gently, try every bite, and chew thoroughly.

Planning your meals in advance

Do not encourage yourself to fall to a meal without realizing what you have and without some food or ingredients.

Plan the meal and shop for that for your week. You will do so regularly because you have the chance to buy every day. And you know what supplies you need and eventually don't purchase more (which you might be tempted to eat). Test what you're going to have for every meal every morning. And if a meal requires pre-preparation, such as soaking beans or frosting, make sure you do so in advance instead of waiting when the food is perfect.

If you don't prepare ahead and are starving ravenously, you would be tented to grab the first item you can find (a bag of chips and a piece of cheese) or go out for pizza.

How safe and low-calorie the food depends on whether you prepare it as well as on the ingredients.

Healthy cooking methods do not have to be involved and developed; they can be hassle-free. Tips for healthy food preparation if you want to lose weight: steam or microwave your vegetables to store more nutrients so that you don't give them extra fat.

Boil the whites, or scramble them; don't cook them. The microwave is capable of making scrambled eggs with a little milk and black pepper. Cook until just before finished, even after removing them from the microwave, they start to cook.

Bake meat or grill and pour the fat away.

Grill them and then place them on paper towels to blot the excess melted fat while frying relatively fatty meat such as bacon or sausages.

Let it go cold when creating a saucepan or stew with fat on it, scrape the solidified fat that exists on top of it, and then heat again.

When making gravy, don't use beef juices that have a lot of fat.

Create your dressing with a little butter, spices, citrus juice, and balsamic vinegar. In this case, you should be assured that in calories, it is much smaller than in-store dressing.

Cover the Mediterranean vegetables and potatoes and roast in the oven with a little olive oil. You may also include thin garlic, pepper, and herbs.

Scientists are continuing to find out about the benefits of exercise, from decreasing the risk of heart disease and osteoporosis to making you happier. It makes you lose calories, but also reduces the tolerance to insulin in PCOS workouts, which gives the bonus of healthier skin, lowers hair loss, decreases the chance of diabetes and increases fertility.

Talk before you start any kind of exercise routine to your doctor; he will probably be enthusiastic about the idea, but he can give you certain specific tips on how to start and what to do or not when you start. While the doctor would not necessarily ban exercise entirely for medical purposes, he may recommend beginning simple workouts gradually, rather than diving straight into half-marathon preparation.

Weight is the contrast between the calories you eat less the calories you lose. The energy-out component of the equation is exercise; the food you consume is the power-in portion. If energy is higher than power, you lose weight.

The body uses two types of fuel (which is the nutrition side): the restful metabolic rate is the nutrition you consume only from holding you alive. Food digestion, breathing, and thinking use energy. You use this energy when you are involved or just sitting on the sofa all day long. The basic metabolic rate is named by medical experts.

During the day, the activity level is the strength you use to drive about. That contains the resources you need to do your duties, go to the bus stop, wash your teeth, etc. ... and all the support that you need to work out formally.

You have not much influence over the specific metabolic rate, but you have a great deal of power over the degree of exercise. Ideally, the fitness program will involve organized workout – a structured task you perform daily over a specified period – plus normal movement during the day.

Compared to only 30 years earlier, people are getting more exercise in the gym today and fewer in their everyday lives. Researchers believe that the regular lack of exercise is at least one explanation for the dramatic rise in obesity. Going to the gym is beneficial for fitness and fat consumption, but elevated rates of practice go above many hours a week. Keeping busy all day allows you to eat calories more than a quick, fast burst of exercise and nothing else.

And how much-organized training will you do regularly?

By the Centers for Disease Control, it is suggested 150 minutes of physical exercise with a mild intensity such as fast walking per week can be helpful. This degree of training can help to compensate for the steady increase in weight that women gain over time.

Practice two days a week for muscle building, utilizing all significant muscle groups such as thighs, arms, neck, belly, stomach, shoulders, and division.

Exercise can be something continuous, like fast biking, planting a yard, mowing the grass (with a mower), swimming or cycling. E.g., when you perform a reasonably vigorous workout for 30 to 35 minutes (such as jogging or cycling), you lose about an extra 300 calories each day. Five days a week should give you a 1500 calorie-per-week shortfall and would reduce your diet from about half a pound a week.

2.2 Workout to Fight PCOS

Being physically active can help reduce much of the effects of PCOS primarily by reducing the tolerance to insulin.

Some tolerance to insulin exists in muscle tissue. Because the muscle tissue cannot efficiently utilize insulin, the pancreas must inject more insulin before it can begin to function. Being mentally inactive only exacerbates addition to insulin. Thus, you get other advantages from doing the physical activity: rendering the body more responsive to the effects of insulin, thereby consuming fewer insulin.

You raise the pace at which glucose is absorbed (to help create muscle energy). This needs less insulin to reduce blood sugar rates.

Reduced insulin concentrations contribute to a more stable menstrual period and hence increased fertility. PCOS signs such as acne and hirsutism reduce. The likelihood of having type 2 diabetes is raised by PCOS. Increasing your amount of fitness (even if you don't lose weight actually) will harm you.

Accumulating fat is a recognized PCOS side effect around the abdomen. Abdominal fat raises the chance of insulin resistance and all the related PCOS symptoms. Data suggests that exercise will tend to reduce the large cell size near the waistline, rather than diet alone.

When obese people were offered a calories-cutting scheme alone or diet plus exercise, those who were exercised displayed reduced fat cells across the abdomen. All types, though, trimmed almost the same quantity of hip cells. The waist was aimed — the most hazardous location to hold fat.

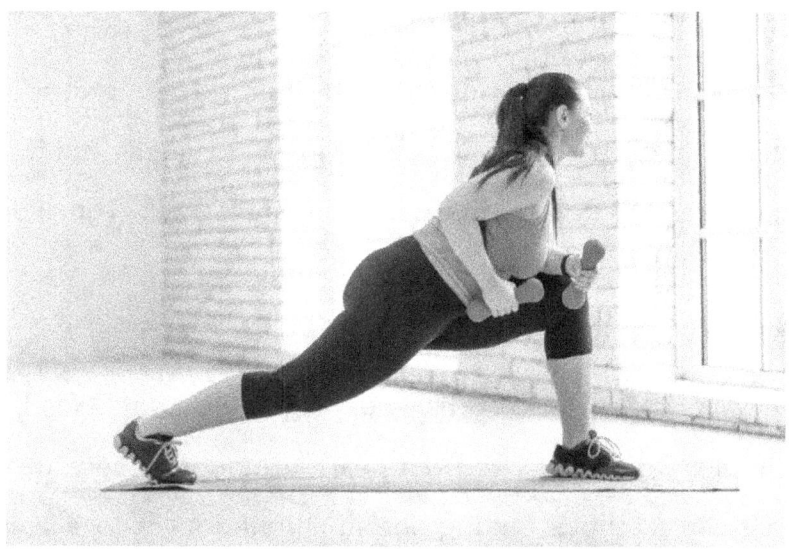

Ground Rules before You Start

Do not necessarily take the preparation and study for a new workout program. Failure to prepare and not to talk about your goals objectively is part of why lifestyle improvements always do not remain there.

If diagnosed with a chronic disorder such as PCOS and are overweight, notify the doctor whether you decide to attend a school or do further taxation exercises. Perhaps she would like to search the heart and lungs. If you have issues with your joint or are fat, your doctor can first recommend that you stop any workouts.

Sadly, 50% of people beginning a training program drop out within six months, especially if they are overweight. But if you will manage to train more than six months back, you would have established a pattern that would be more likely to maintain in the long term.

Remember the following as you pick a workout: Heed the recommendation of your health care provider. If he wants to skip such activities, taking certain limitations into account, think seriously about how much you will be working out. Don't hinder your performance by attempting too fast.

Plan the regular workout like cycling rather than driving the ride. This allows you to stay involved all day and improves the likelihood you can stick with it. After all, you would go home if you walked to the supermarket!

Have the children in your work. Holding the children socially healthy always has psychological advantages for them. Go swimming or take long walks for relaxing and exercise as a team. If your thing is professional sports, enter a coordinated squad of attractions. Golf is also a sport – drop the cart at the course! If you want a company when exercise, pick fitness courses or social activities for family or mates.

You can exercise for free or pay for lessons at school. You should mix and match — go to college twice a week and perform a workout DVD with them at home. Combine fitness and also improve your social life. Go to the party and meet a few new friends. Many colleges or adult education centers provide small dance courses. Know yourself and prepare by entering a class in martial arts like Tae Kwan Do or Kickboxing. Such practices would undoubtedly boost the heart rate! When it comes to inspiration, try investing in a personal trainer. You can be encouraged to keep moving if you realize you've wasted the gas. If you like to exercise and it is in your everyday life, you are far more likely to get routine physical activity.

Today, whenever practicable, physical exercise will be performed on at least five weekdays for at least 30 minutes a day, to gain the maximum benefits of becoming involved and that the effects of PCOS. If you want you can perform aerobics in 10 minutes, you don't have to do it for 30 minutes at once. Exercise resistance two or three times a week, but leave a day for each session if necessary or exercise specific muscles while you are practicing on consecutive days. Perform some stability exercises after aerobic preparation. When you consider that soothing, do the Pilates, the T'ai Chi, or the like (see the segment on "Maintenance of stability," later); if you choose, one of them is accessible once a week or every day. Every such exercise has various consequences and advantages. Ideally, these three forms of workout are to be incorporated during the week.

Aerobic exercise

One of the meanings is "sustained activity that incorporates broad muscle groups and puts cardiovascular demands." In other terms, the type of workout beats the heart and leaves you a little short of breath.

The aerobic activity provides the following benefits if you have PCOS: It strengthens the heart and lung function. It reduces insulin and addiction to insulin. It lowers blood sugar. It helps to lower blood pressure. It improves the mood. It accelerates your metabolism and enables you to eat more calories both after and during exercise. Every workout that raises the pulse and heart rhythm and warms up can be considered cardiovascular, like cycling, jogging, biking, digging, and dancing. Experts suggest that you perform any physical exercise at least 30 minutes five days a week. You may want to proceed gradually and see your doctor before you continue if you haven't performed some aerobic workouts for a while.

If it is challenging to find the time to perform a decent half-hour aerobic workout, it is ideal to do so in ten minutes. Driving quickly to the bus stop, wandering about at lunchtime, pulling your strawberry, or moving the vacuum cleaner through the house briskly, add up about ten minutes.

Cheap, quick, and good for you to move. If you have PCOS and have excess weight, walking is a perfect workout that will not bother the joints too much. Plus, walking is the most popular workout people do when they get older. A routine walking regimen can carry some of the benefits that you have to offer: reduced rest heart rate (a sign of general health). Decreased blood pressure Calorie intake Reduced stress rates Improved muscle tone Weight loss Reduced heart attack or stroke risk. There isn't any room or a specific spot to do it. Including though you fly, you should continue your fitness routine.

Experts suggest that you operate three or four days a week for around 45 minutes. That should be the goal, not anything you do automatically. The watchwords are shorter distances and less time when you launch. Weight running, weight-machine use, and resistance band exercises are used in the strength exercise. Technically, strength exercise simply involves fighting against mass, energy, or momentum. Resistance exercise has these advantages: it improves strength, muscle capacity, and body size. It helps to raise the metabolic rate and hence the fat-burning ability. It is believed that muscle tissue is up to 70 times more metabolically active than fat — quite relevant if you have PCOS!

It helps to reduce the tolerance to insulin, which is necessary for raising PCOS symptoms. This may also decrease blood pressure, which in PCOS continues to be higher. This tends to reduce osteoporosis since bones are hardened by weight and the strength of stiff muscles.

It tends to account for lower back discomfort and other body issues while increases the health and equilibrium. It leaves the muscles primed for action and trained. With muscle power and flexibility, it appears to be "used or discarded." The study has demonstrated that nearly any advantage of resistance exercise is gained in two training sessions of 15-20 minutes a week. Responsive resistance training involves precise, coordinated movements in any major muscle group and does not allow hefty weights to be used. You may integrate this style of workout into the fitness regimen in many respects. This is simple and safe to use your body weight, for example, bent-knee sit-ups or stomach twists, push-ups, and chin-ups. However, you have to attach things like bands of resistance or free weights to deal with your body weight.

Use resistance bands

These devices are lightweight and can be modified for several exercise sessions. E.g., to focus on the biceps, you step on the drum, keep up, and down the other end of your hand. The bands offer constant tension during a cycle, unlike free weights. However, groups are not as massive on the muscle as a free weight, which suggests that they are the best fit for soft firming and toning. Free weights like dumbbells or barbells should be used to work on anybody's muscle. You typically require a workout facility or a variety of weights at home. Beginners may use everyday kitchen objects, such as a few soup cans, for dumbbells. Don't drop them on your foot. Don't drop them on your foot!

Weight devices: Weight devices have adjustable seats with handles connected to either mechanical or weight. For beginners, weight machines are useful because they direct the activity and maintain proper form. But a weight machine cannot always be calibrated to match the body size and shape.

Many health experts recommend that you weigh 8 to 12 inches. Then you may replay the entire package 2-3 times.

Wait 24 to 48 hours for a similar group of muscles in resistance training sessions. However, during the time, you will focus on a particular group of muscles.

Maintaining flexibility

Being smooth and agile strengthens the posture and equilibrium and allows you to hold the entire body is going. Although it's not necessary to aid with PCOS symptoms, being versatile is part of the overall kit that makes you look better and feel better.

Stretching you will still reach your muscles before and during a workout, no matter whether you are performing strength training, cardiovascular fitness, or both, to stop stiffening up muscles and joints. Two of the benefits of relaxing are: it increases overall health. Mental and physical stimulation may be improved. The possibility of damage to limbs, muscles, and tendons may be familiar. It helps avoid or reduce muscle soreness. It helps to improve flexibility by stimulating chemical development, which lubricates joints. The intensity of the traumatic menstruation may also be accessible.

Never drive yourself into a stretch or jump through it; just let your body recover, or yourself injure. Use guidance again from a professional exercise coach or a decent DVD (or try out Dependency for Dummies, Madeleine Lewis [Wiley], by Larine Chabot). If you suffer from fractures, muscle, or joint issues, obtains medical assistance before you start.

Unlike exercise usage, it serves to hold the different joints in the body rigid to inform them of the motions they will be able to produce.

Many classes are provided with a high degree of flexibility like Yoga, which helps you to regulate your body and mind and to strengthen your breathing and concentrate your body's balance Pilates: a type of training which aims to build your body's consciousness, to improve posture and stability, and to enhance flexibility and ease of movement T'ai C. If you have PCOS, they are a gentle way to begin the workout without getting stressed out and discouraged. When you consider exercising a bit harder and even enjoyable, add more strenuous workouts to affect PCOS symptoms.

Follow the food recommendations in this book to support your PCOS. There you will get some simple tips to optimize the advantages of physical exercise when consuming a healthy PCOS diet: consume a broad range of foods and make sure the body gets enough of the meals at its best. Do so in general, so stop drinking before or during a workout if you consume alcohol. Make sure that before and during the exercise, you are well hydrated. Should not fail to consume enough fluids during a workout to account for the moisture loss in sweat. Eat several low-GI carbohydrates. As the energy release from low to medium-GI foods is slower, this form of food will allow you to exercise faster without steam running out. Feed modest protein numbers. Feed two parts of the fish a week, one oily. Don't perform a full stomach exercise right after a nice meal. If you exercise every day, enjoy smaller main meals and treats to boost your energy levels.

Pregnancy Exercise

Here are a few essential tips on pregnancy exercise. Both women, irrespective of whether or not they have PCOS, provide this advice: When you have become physically active previous to becoming pregnant, continuity of the preparation is excellent, so long as the workout is reasonably demanding and does not reach 30 to 40 minutes.

Marathons are currently out racing. Avoid exercise, which requires intensive training for a long time. Exercising aerobically 3 or 4 days a week cannot be more than 30 or 40 minutes a week during pregnancy. It is especially crucial if you should not have a weight-bearing workout (although you may want to stick to a stationary cycle in late pregnancy, so you are not as prone to fall). In the third section, stop workouts that lay flat on your stomach. As long as you learn that you are breastfeeding, confirm with your doctor if the workout is all right. As a PCOS user, you might have had miscarriage problems in the past. Tell your surgeon what exercises you should perform and what you can refrain from. Before exercising, you will have the difference between an enthusiastic (perhaps even peppy) workout and a bored look-to-your-watch-each-five-minute workout. Follow these basic principles to fuel your preparation.

Early morning workouts

When you prefer early workouts, so you should put on anything to stop getting dizzy and famished (before the body has a chance to protest). Give ample room to eat the meal to prevent diarrhea or cramping. Say this: If you work out within an hour of waking up, eat 200 to 300 calories before exercise. Keep the fat intake minimal, as fat can stay in the stomach for some time, wait until it is digested, and feel miserable while you work out. Healthy food options include whole-grain cereals, raisins, bananas, or mixed fruit and milk-based beverages in the early morning classroom. Or grab a few pieces of full-grain bread with mashed banana and some peanut butter.

Lunchtime workouts

At lunchtime, it is just a vague recollection for breakfast. A low GI, fat carbohydrate-rich snack one or two hours before the exercise will reduce nausea and exhaustion throughout the lunchtime exercise.

A milkshake, whole-grain crackers with peanut butter or hummus, yogurt, berries (fresh or dried), or a little bowl of low GI grain would be an excellent option. Make sure, after your workout, and you consume a healthy meal. The workday's over, you're on the road to the gym, and you're hungry. Will the steering wheel transform the car suddenly into the closest fast-food restaurant? Since lunch has been around for a long time and the body's full of food. You ought to obey the same guidelines for launchers: Get a low GI, low-fat snack that is high with carbs one or two hours before your exercise. And then enjoy a nutritious meal.

When you stop training, any of the calories that you consumed will be absorbed; when you exercised hard, the glycogen levels are likely to be small and need to be depleted.

Glycogen is a readily available fuel supply for your body and gradually absorbs glucose during exercise. When the glycogen stores are not depleted (which are contained in the liver and muscles), that ensures you have too little room for the next nutrition supply.

After work workout

Be sure your after-work out diet is a decent source of carbohydrates to boost your glycogen stores. With any nutrition, the body may strengthen the capacity to regenerate glycogen. Don't wait too long after exercising until you take a lunch or a snack, or you can be completely energy-less.

CHAPTER 3: INSULIN RESISTANCE DIET AND PCOS

Most people have polycystic ovarian syndrome (PCOS) or high insulin. High insulin is both a sign of PCOS and an underlying physiological engine. Insulin resistance testing can help remove other conditions often misdiagnosed because PCOS polycystic ovarian syndrome sounds like it's just an ovary's disease. Although PCOS is an endocrine and metabolic disease of the entire body and is strongly linked to insulin tolerance, it can involve ovaries and ovulation.

The enzyme lepton rises slightly when feeding under usual circumstances. This activates the liver and muscles to take blood sugar and convert it into electricity. Which then allows blood sugar to decrease, accompanied by insulin? Sugar and insulin are ordinary in a fasting blood check for good insulin sensitivity.

Blood sugar may be natural with insulin tolerance, but insulin is high. Why? Why? Since the pancreas must generate more and more insulin to get out the post. Excessive insulin induces swelling, and weight gain. Type 2 diabetes and heart failure can also occur. A natural biochemical cause of PCOS Insulin tolerance is too much insulin, an integral characteristic of both obese and lean PCOS. This is observed in 70-95% of persons with heavy PCOS and 30-75% of persons with thin PCOS.

Fast insulin is not only a PCOS sign but also a pioneer in the disease. High insulin can induce ovulation and excess testosterone in the ovaries.

One research showed that a growing prevalence of PCOS corresponds with a rise in obesity and weight gain over the last decade. As a clinic that prescribes diet and natural therapies for PCOS, we need to validate insulin resistance with a blood check such as fasting insulin, Home-IR index or a 2-hour insulin glucose challenge measurement, which is part of a paper identified as a "galloping rise in PCOS" in conjunction with the increasing prevalence in type 2 diabetes. Traditional insulin resistance guidelines include weight loss, physical workouts, and diabetic medication. Training in resistance may also be successful, but more work is required.

Another standardized therapy for PCOS is oral contraception, although it can conflict with sugar management and insulin tolerance to PCOS. The association between PCOS, insulin resistance, and oral contraceptive pills has been referred to as a 'real medical issue' which requires more study.

Fructose itself is not a problem; it can only inflict damage by a significant volume. For example, low doses of fruit fructose do not induce insulin resistance and are advantageous for insulin sensitivity and safety. Desserts, soft drinks, and fruit juice with high dose fructose have a somewhat different effect. "There is a basic biochemical distinction in the way smaller and bigger sugar is handled in the body," one researcher clarified. At large doses, fructose can disrupt natural digestion processes in the small intestine, which may contribute to inflammation, which insulin sensitivity in the liver. More analysis is expected here.

Inositol is an insulin carrier that should be used as a dietary substitute (my-inositol that di-chirp inositol). A review of 10 randomized studies in 2018 showed that inositol substantially enhanced insulin resistance markers and "appeared to control menstrual cycles, promote ovulation, and cause metabolic improvements in polycystic ovary syndrome." The dosage used in most controlled trials ranged between 1.2 and 4 grams a day. Magnesium is my second favorite insulin resistance drug as it helps to address the prevalent subclinical magnesium deficiency reported by sure researchers being responsible for insulin resistance and cardiac failure. Magnesium deficiency impacts at least one-third of individuals and potentially higher and cannot be detected by a blood test quickly or accurately.

The latest meta-analysis has suggested that magnesium supplementation is beneficial for the treatment of insulin resistance in people with magnesium deficiency, and a recent review has shown that magnesium, zinc, calcium, and vitamin D co-supplementation has increased PCOS insulin metabolism.

3.1 Coping with Insulin Resistance and Its Effects

Insulin plays a crucial role in glucose absorption into cells, where it can be used for energy. Insulin is such an active hormone that it cannot contribute to hyperglycemia (high rates of glucose) and death. When cells build a tolerance to insulin, they no longer respond to insulin release by taking glucose. This contributes to elevated amounts of glucose, which in turn has other unintended health consequences.

In this segment, we address the production of insulin resistance, its impact on health, and, most significantly, how you can overcome it.

Resistance to insulin is a progressive disorder that triggers the bulk of PCOS symptoms. The susceptibility to insulin is not rare – it affects around 3% of individuals. The pancreas produces insulin in the natural metabolic cycle as a consequence of food consumption and glucose presence in the bloodstream. For a variety of factors, this phase is terrible in terms of insulin tolerance. The problem as to why insulin resistance firstly occurs is complicated. Nevertheless, the following factors lead to insulin resistance: genetics: specific genes that lead to insulin resistance and Type 2 diabetes.

Overweight: In fact, the weight that builds up about the hips is correlated with insulin resistance.

Abnormal lipids: Increased triglyceride and cholesterol rates in the blood may raise the likelihood of insulin resistance.

High blood pressure: Elevated blood pressure scientifically labeled hypertension leads to the production of tolerance to insulin.

High serum cortisol rates: fatigue and heavy meat consumption are two sources of elevated levels of cortisol. Cortisol counteracts hormone that adds to the tolerance to the hormone.

Resistance to insulin is a significant predictor of the possibility of diabetes type 2. When blood sugar rates are elevated, and diabetes is established, several cells containing insulin could already have been killed in the pancreas. Insulin resistance early detection and care before irrevocably damaged cells generating insulin can postpone or avoid the onset of type 2 diabetes.

The major problem with the susceptibility to insulin is the possible occurrence of type 2 diabetes. Easy to feed, lose weight, and exercise are ways to avoid insulin tolerance from diabetes.

If you believe improvements to nutrition and exercise cannot improve, chew on these facts: consume fewer calories in days, and before you lose weight, much less insulin resistance.

- Losing between 10 and 20 pounds has a significant impact on blood glucose rates.

- Losing 16% of body weight improves the production of glucose by 100%.

- Exercise will improve the sensitivity to insulin for up to 16 hours after the test.

3.2 The Glycemic Index and Diet

A Glycemic Index Diet is a diet focused on how foods affect the levels of blood sugar.

The glycemic index is a system by which carbohydrate-containing foods are distributed according to how much blood sugar each meal increases. The glycemic index is not a diet plan by nature, but one of many ways of controlling food choices – including calorie counting or carbon counting.

The term "glycemic index diet" typically refers to a specific diet that uses the index for food planning as a primary or only guide. Unlike some other programs, for weight loss or weight maintenance, a glycemic index diet does not automatically dictate portion sizes or the optimum amount of calories or carbs or fats.

Many typical marketing diets, diet books and diet websites, including the Zone Diet, Sugar Busters, and the Slow Carb Diet, are focused on glycemic indexes.

A glycemic index (GI) diet is designed to feed carbohydrate-containing foods less likely to cause significant increases in blood sugar levels. Diet may be a way of losing weight and avoiding chronic obesity-related diseases such as diabetes and cardiovascular disease.

You can decide to follow the GI diet if:

- You want to lose weight or maintain your healthy weight
- You need support in preparing and eating healthier meals
- You need help managing blood sugar levels in your diabetes treatment plan.

However, by eating a healthy diet, maintaining a healthy weight, and having enough exercise, you can obtain the same health benefits.

Before you start a weight loss diet, consult with your doctor or healthcare provider, particularly if you have any health conditions like diabetes.

The GI theory was first developed as a method to guide food choices for diabetes patients. Sydney University Glycemic Index Testing Facilities in Sydney, Australia, operates a regional GI database. The report contains the results of studies carried out there and in other research centers worldwide.

A detailed description of carbohydrates, blood sugar, and GI values is essential for glycemic index diets.

Carbohydrates or carbs are a kind of food nutrient. The three fundamental types are sugar, starch, and fiber. When you eat or drink with carbs, the sugars and starches in your body become a form of sugar called glucose, the principal source of cellular energy. Fiber moves undigested through your body.

Two essential hormones in your pancreas help to control blood glucose. Glucose is transferred from your blood into your cells by the hormone insulin. The glucagon hormone helps release your liver glucose if your blood sugar (blood glucose) is weak. This cycle allows the body to keep fueling and maintains an average blood glucose level.

Different forms of carbohydrate food have an influence on how easily your body digests and how easily your bloodstream absorbs glucose.

There are various methods of research to give a GI value to food. The figure is usually based on how much blood glucose a food product increases relative to how much pure blood glucose raises.

- Low GI values: 1 to 55
- Medium gig: 56 to 69
- High gig I values: 70 and higher

So the comparison of these values will help to make healthy food choices. An English muffin made from white wheat flour, for example, has a GI value of 77. The GI value of a full wheat English muffin is 45.

One drawback of GI values is that it does not represent the likely amount of food you are consuming.

For example, watermelon has a GI of 80, which means that this is to be avoided in the food category. But in a standard section, watermelon has relatively few digestible carbohydrates. In other words, you will consume a lot of melons to increase your blood glucose levels dramatically.

To deal with this issue, researchers have introduced the concept of glycemic load (GL), a numerical value indicating changes in blood glucose levels when a healthy portion of the food is taken. For example, a 4, 2-ounce piece of watermelon (120 grams, or 3/4 cups) has a GL of 5, which is a healthy food option. A 2.8-ounce part (80-g or 2/3-cup) of raw carrots has a GL value of 2 for comparison.

The GI values table at Sydney University also contains GL values.

- Low GL: 1 to 10
- Medium GL: 11 to 19
- high GL: 20 or more

A GI value doesn't tell us much about any other nutritional details. For instance, whole milk has a GI value of 31 and a GL value of 4 for a serving of 1 task (250 mm). However, due to its high-fat content, whole milk is not the safest way to control weight loss or weight gain.

The published GI database is not a complete food list, but a list of the foods studied. There are other balanced foods, not in the database, with low GI values.

Many factors are influencing the GI value of any food item, including how it is cooked, processed, and what other foods are consumed at the same time.

A selection of GI values for the same foods may also be identified, and some may argue that it is an inaccurate guide to the determination of food choices.

A GI diet generally prescribes foods with low values.

- Green vegetables, most fruit, essential carrots, kidney beans, chickpeas, lentils and cereals for breakfast bran
- sweet-grain, banana, raw pineapple, raisin, cereal for oat breakfast and multigrain, oat bran or rye bread
- white rice, white bread, and potatoes Commercial

GI Diets can include foods with low, middle, and high GI values. Foods with a low GI are usually digested and consumed relatively slowly, whereas foods with high GI values are easily absorbed.

Commercial GI diets have various portion size requirements as well as protein and fat intake.

Studies of the effects of GI diets have provided mixed outcomes, depending on the health goals.

The results of a 16-year study that tracked the diets of 120,000 men and women were published in 2015. Researchers found that processed grains, starches, and sugar are related to more significant weight gain in foods with high GL.

Many studies indicate that a low GI diet can also lead to weight loss and weight loss. Nevertheless, evidence from another study shows a vast number of different GI values for the same foods. This spectrum of variation in GI values is an unreliable guide to food choices.

Studies show that the total carbohydrate in food is typically a better indicator than the GI of blood glucose reaction.

Blood glucose control: Based on the study, the easiest way for most people with diabetes to regulate blood glucose is to count carbohydrates.

Some clinical trials have shown that a low-GI diet may enable people who have diabetes to regulate their blood glucose, but the results found may be due to low calorie, high fiber levels of the foods given in the research.

These foods may lead to lower total cholesterol as well as low-density lipoproteins (the "poor" cholesterol) — especially when a low-GI diet is coupled with an increase in food fiber — have shown to be relatively consistent in cholesterol testing. Foods with low to moderate GIs such as fruits, vegetables, and whole grains are typically healthy fiber sources.

Appetite regulation: One low-GI diet effect hypothesis is appetite management. It is believed that GI food induces a rapid rise in blood glucose, a quick response to insulin, and then an early return to starvation. Low-GI foods, in effect, can postpone hunger feelings. Clinical trials have shown mixed findings for this theory.

Often, if a low-GI diet suppresses appetite, it could be a long-term impact on people to consume less and control their weight more effectively. However, long-term clinical work does not show this impact.

You need to eat as many calories as you consume in order to maintain your current weight. You have to eat more calories than you consume to lose weight. The best way to achieve weight loss is to incorporate calorie restriction and improve physical activity and exercise.

You can control your weight by selecting foods based on a glycemic index or glycemic load values, as many items that need to be included in a balanced, low-fat, organic diet with minimally-processed foods – grain products, fruits, vegetables, and low-fat dairy products – are low GI.

Some people will need to use a commercial low GI diet to help them make better decisions for a healthier diet. However, researchers who manage the GI database warn to consider the "glycemic index" and other nutritional factors such as calories, fat, protein, vitamins, and other nutrients.

3.3 What Is Insulin Resistance Diet?

As our insulin resistance's function and impact continue to increase, we become more and more conscious of diseases that are affected by insulin impaired behavior. The degree to which insulin affects these conditions can vary. However, influences that reduce insulin resistance also have a positive effect on symptoms and outcomes. At the same time, there is still a clear indication that the underlying cause of insulin resistance is closely associated with the sophisticated collection of defense and repair mechanisms known as inflammation.

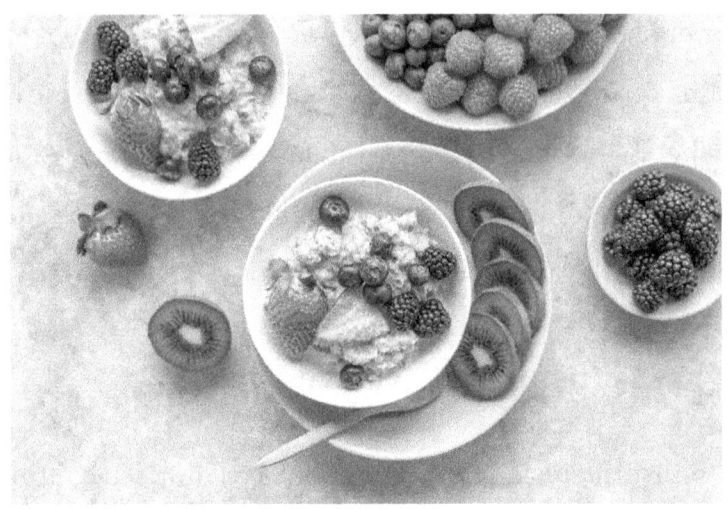

PCOS is one of the disorders involving concurrent metabolic and endocrine etiologies, and insulin resistance is a prevalent factor in most cases. In reproductive women, PCOS is the most common endocrine condition, but many women suffer from PCOS and its different manifestations long before they are diagnosed formally. As a result, they suffer from persistent, debilitating symptoms and fertility issues that are physically and emotionally very difficult. A diagnosis of PCOS is mostly based on fertility and the reproductive system. However, the metabolic aspect of this syndrome is essential for both short-term and long-term health and productivity.

Although we discuss the role of insulin and inflammation as it relates to PCOS, and the well-formulated ketogenic diet and its known effects on the resistance and inflammation of insulin that also benefit some women suffering from this syndrome.

PCOS is a cluster of symptoms that differ from woman to woman. Any of these signs are mild, unpleasant, extreme and irregular cycles of the menstrual, increased body hair, dark skin patches, mood disorder, and infertility. There are several PCOS phenotypes and diagnostic criteria for PCOS, but women with PCOS usually have at least two of the three key characteristics of:

- Excess of androgen (can occur as body hair increased)
- Chronic oligo/anovulation (can occur as absent or abnormal periods of the menstruation)
- The involvement of polycystic ovaries at the diagnosis time.

However, two specific components are underlying these critical features of several metabolic diseases: insulin resistance and inflammation.

While not a part of official diagnostic criteria, the signs of PCOS and another metabolism such as type 2 diabetes (T2D), obesity, dyslipidemias, alcoholic fatty liver disease (NAFLD) are not only affected by insulin resistance and inflammation but also by the relationship of PCOS to other metabolic disorders. Indeed, women without PCOS have a 2-4 times higher risk of prediabetes, T2D, gestational diabetes, and obesity, which may potentially lead to an increased risk of cardiovascular and endometrial cancers.

PCOS's metabolic and hormonal signals frequently intensify a vicious cycle that exacerbates symptoms. Chronically elevated insulin, which further sends signals to the ovaries to increase androgen production, excess androgens also contribute to a higher abdominal pain of fat, and increased abdominal fat then, aggravates inflammation and insulin resistance, thereby continuing the life cycle. PCOS and its metabolic risks should, therefore, be viewed in a broader sense of health outside of female fertility.

The insulin resistance and reduced tolerance to glucose are present in a significant proportion (ranging from 44 to 70 percent) of women with PCOS. The resistance to insulin is a significant contributor to metabolic disorders and a catalyst for PCOS pathogenesis. Therefore, hyperinsulinemia, hyperglycemia, and elevated oxidative stress, usually associated with insulin deregulation, all contribute to the disease. It is not entirely understood how insulin deregulation takes place in this condition but is possibly due to impaired insulin suppression and receptor activity leading to increased insulin secretion and reduced liver clearance. One consequence of this continuous insulin rise is a higher signal for the ovaries and an improved development of androgen.

Post-prandial or post-meal dysglycemia in PCOS is more common than rapid dysglycemia commonly seen in diabetes. This will help to boost the indicator of prediabetes and T2D in these patients through the existence of impaired glucose tolerance (IGT). An oral glucose tolerance test (OGTT) is considered a more appropriate test for the identification of prediabetes or T2D risk in females with PCOS than HbA1c. Because of the impact of insulin resistance in PCOS, conventional therapies include insulin-sensitizing medicines, including metformin. Dietary adjustments and exercise are often prescribed to increase insulin sensitivity, but sometimes as vague and undescribed medications, if they are approved.

Insulin signaling has a strong interwoven relationship with inflammation, known to affect fertility and weight gain. Inflammation impairs glucose tolerance and insulin function, and it may be one of the connections between hyperandrogenism, insulin resistance, and PCOS abdominal obesity. Inflammation is possible to some degree involved in the root causes of many chronic diseases, and the PCOS is not an exception. Inflammatory markers such as CRP, IL-6, White

Blood Cell Count (WBC), and TNF-a are increased in PCOS patients and may raise the risk of age-old health complications (3, 4). These inflammatory factors, such as WBC, CRP, and TNF-a, are also associated with increased risk for T2D and cardiovascular disease.

There are many causes of this increased PCOS inflammation. Visceral fatty adipose tissue accumulates strong insulin resistance and swelling in the abdomen and around the organs and contains many proinflammatory cytokines and adipocytes. These adipocytokines play a part in cardiovascular risk factors such as dyslipidemia and endothelial dysfunction. Inflammation linked to excess central fat accumulation can also be a significant factor in ovarian dysfunction, and inflammation can lead to hyperandrogenism. Excess inflammation can be managed generally by using anti-inflammatory agents. Many of these medicines target certain bioactive compounds (e.g., TNF-a, IL1-b) in the inflammatory system, which can cause side effects such as immune suppression. Low carbohydrate and well-formulated ketogenic diets, but without compromised immune response or other specific factors of anti-inflammatory drugs, have been demonstrated to minimize the number of many inflammatory biomarkers like CRP and WBC.

PCOS / The metabolic symptoms of PCOS do not shock that the predominance of prediabetic and T2D in patients with PCOS is more significant than age and weight-matched women without PCOS (15). There has been some kind of chicken or egg dispute about what first occurs in PCOS, inflammation.

The connection to Dyslipidemia, Obeticism and Type 2 Diabetes

Due to the absorption of PCOS, many patients may have signs of dyslipidemia irrespective of diabetes or high blood pressure. About age and weight-matched controls, studies reported more elevated triglycerides and non-HDL cholesterol as well as lower HDD in women with PCOS. Obesity will intensify the complication risk. However, in most women with PCOS, some degree of insulin resistance is observed regardless of BMI. As insulin resistance is essential for the development of prediabetes and T2D, the risk of these conditions is rising with PCOS. Risk identification can help to identify and avoid problems associated with these conditions.

The potentials of a well-formulated Ketogenic diet on PCOS

A well-formulated Ketogenic diet (WFKD) is reversed, inflammation reduced, and weight loss facilitated. Consequently, without the side effects of prescription medication, women can be able to use a WFKD to boost many necessary signals that lead to PCOS.

Women with PCOS appear to experience oxidative stress in response to the ingestion of glucose. To exacerbate the issue, the characteristic hyperandrogenism of the syndrome tends to enhance the inflammatory response to glucose. Reducing carbohydrates with WFKD increases the sensitivity to insulin, and the subsequent reduction of chronically elevated insulin will affect the production and signaling of androgen in the ovaries. Ketones (specifically beta-hydroxybutyrate (BOHB)) are not only used for fuel but also have antioxidant effects. You et al. stated that the function of a significant inflammatory control gene is also controlled by BOHB. This offers a multi-level solution to squash inflammation. During painful periods and inflammation, chronic low-grade inflammation may reduce the quality of life and fertility.

The status of the hormone is also critical for fertility concerns. The WFKD can boost the hormonal profile of women with PCOS and increase their chances of pregnancy in two small studies. The participants who were able to complete the study showed substantial weight loss and improvements in the percent of free testosterone, LH / FSH (luteinizing hormone / follicle-stimulating hormone) and fasting insulin in the 24-

week procedure using ketogenic diet in which 11 females with PCOS were instructed to reduce carbohydrates to less than twenty grams per day. And of these five completers, two were planned successfully without the use of fertility medicines. In the study of 8 PCOS patients, four were able to adopt the diet, 2 of whom were born without medically induced ovulation, and recommended a calorie-restricted ketogenic diet for six months.

It should be noted that these two pilot studies were minimal and unrandomized. That said, four out of nine patients in these two trials were promising to sustain a ketogenic diet developed by natural means for six months (40%-50% of success rates). This seems to be comparable to the possible design rates of 30-40 percent in 5 monthly pharmaceutical ovulation cycles. Finally, environmental and behavioral variables must also be taken into consideration in PCOS care. Lower satiety and higher sweet cravings have been identified in women with PCOS and are likely to lead to weight gain. The issues with "dieting" were well known, but for those living with nutritional ketosis, a calorically suitable, well-designed ketogenic diet has been proven to increase satiety. While these characteristics are contradictory to many government recommendations, the continuously rising number of research projects supports the use of restricted carbohydrates and increasing dietary fat for enhancing insulin sensitivity and reducing inflammation.

PCOS is typically associated with increased inflammation and insulin resistance, and a WFKD has shown that both of these have potent effects. And in contrast to most medications, a WFKD has few if any permanent side-effects that are more than balanced by weight improvements, blood pressure, blood glucose control, and dyslipidemia. But what are the consequences for women seeking to conceive while adopting a ketogenic diet? Despite the two small published studies that indicate that 40-50 percent of women with PCOS will develop a natural definition following a ketogenic diet, there are no significant studies that show the safety of carrying a pregnancy until the end when following a WFKD. The healthcare practice is, therefore, to recommend that a ketogenic diet be stopped if women are pregnant.

Women with PCOS have a high risk for pregnancy, preeclampsia and premature birth (all raised by 1.5 to 2.5) Unfortunately we cannot be motivated by current research given the lack of reliable evidence to balance the risk of continuing with a carbohydrate-restricted diet during pregnancy against the risk of the PCOS-associated complications of a more conventional diet.

PCOS has physical and emotional consequences. While the condition can be different for women, most patients have insulin deregulation and inflammation that lead to the syndrome. Besides this, many patients are not aware of the underlying metabolic issues. Both causes might have a significant impact on insulin and swelling if they treated by a well-formulated ketogenic diet without the side effects associated with pharmaceutical treatments.

3.4 Other Advice for Healthy Eating

Nobody likes rules and rigidity, especially about food. However, if you adopt the low GI diet, keep some stuff in mind: check.png when you eat a car, make sure it's a low GI diet. If it is difficult to find a low-GI food or if you want a change from time to time, use a medium-GI menu.

On a special occasion (or when you go to the house of a friend on dinner and don't want to be rude), sometimes eating high-GI food isn't too much damage. To preserve the safe and low GI of your diet, follow the following tips: for drinks, a nutritious soft drink, tea and coffee (in moderation), or low-calorie hot chocolate. You are using artificial sweeteners to sweeten your hot drink, which will save on empty calories. Also, stop drinking more than one or two alcoholic beverages a day, and stick mostly with food mixers to dry wines or spirits.

Avoid adding salt to food and reduce high-salt food intake. Don't consume too many protein foods like beef, fish, eggs, poultry, and cheese. Two parts of these are okay a day. You are using soy or peas, beans, and lentils as protein choices if you are a vegetarian. These are healthy and low in fat, so even if you are not vegetarian, they're careful to eat. Control your fat intake. Stop frying the food and substitute polyunsaturated fats and oils (such as butter, lard, cookies, biscuits, and pastries). Avoid Tran's fats; this is a product to avoid if you see partly hydrogenated on the bottle.

Seek to get enough calcium for three servings of milk food a day. Apart is one small yogurt tub, 2/3 cup of milk, or 1 ounce of cheese.

Get enough of food fiber. Fiber can give blood sugar regulation over and above the GI effect alone a boost. Seek to get between 25 and 35 grams a day; most Americans just eat about 11 grams a day!

Allow yourself to be served one day, like an ice cream scoop or a low-induced bakery such as a muffin or a small slice of pound cake. Do not take dietary supplements or take alternative treatments without instruction from medically trained health professionals, including doctors or dietitians.

British nutritionists produced a pictorial representation, called the balance of good health, of the components of a balanced diet. The following parts provide you with some other tips to maintain a healthy and low GI diet.

3.5 Taking Medications

PCOS is one of the common hormonal condition in women of reproductive age. PCOS is questionable. Nevertheless, there is no remedy for the disease, and most therapies are meant to relieve the symptoms. Many drugs will undoubtedly help to reduce the symptoms, however, and other medicines are attempting to cure the underlying PCOS cause: the resistance to insulin. In this chapter, we look at available medications and think about the benefits and drawbacks of using them. Several drug groups are used for treating insulin resistance, one of the critical causes of symptoms in the cascade, which can affect PCOS people. Each has various behavior and side effects.

It is reported in 2004, Americans paid over $20 billion on supplements of different kinds. More than 50% of Americans use some sort of dietary supplement per year. There are no restrictions to the forms of over the counter weight loss items, from homeopathic remedies to vitamins, food substitute beverages, and diet bars.

Meal replacement beverages and diet bars, where a dietary supplement substitutes for a meal, are usually the least harmful. Notwithstanding their extravagant claims, most herbs and other supplements provide no significant weight loss.

While many of the more harmful herbs and supplements have now been banned, everywhere, even on the Internet, you can still find that they are for sale. There are also more potentially harmful substances, and even drugs that are not health-dangerous can be detrimental to your pocketbook.

The banned narcotics were based on unsafe medicines such as amphetamines and ephedra (also known as ma hang). Some weight-loss herbs have recently been reported as contributing to liver toxicity.

A recent study in a medical journal reported that the use of performance enhancement and weight loss supplements in the United States is widespread. These medications are the kind athletes use to control their weight and sports skills. However, anyone trying to lose weight may also take them. The book discusses many of the side effects of these supplements, including the knowledge that caffeine-based herbal supplements are especially risky to search for because they can lead to remarkably high blood pressure.

Some of the supplements marketed today are particularly difficult to test as they are not one ingredient but blended. You won't know which herb or medication triggered it if you have an adverse reaction. Many have names that sound very much like prescription medicines.

As over-the-counter supplements sometimes shift, it is challenging to keep a comprehensive list up-to-date. Some of the supplements that were favorite at the time of this writing are Acai: The acai berry, coming from the Brazilian Amazon region, is a high antioxidant berry. Proponents contend that acai is a super food that has weight loss effects and a range of other health advantages.

Chromium: Chromium sold as a pollinate chromium is a popular perennial diet. This mineral will increase the sensitivity to insulin, resulting in weight loss.

Green tea: Green tea fans say that it improves thermogenesis. Green tea contains caffeine, which, even with unpleasant side effects, can speed your metabolism in large amounts.

Hoodia: This African medicine is a cactus-like plant that appears to have strong appetite-suppressive properties that function to make the brain feel complete. Since efficient and safe hoodia limits were not set, it is difficult to know whether or not the product you buy would have any impact.

Yohimbe: A central nervous system stimulant, made of the bark of the evergreen tree, Yohimbe, or the chemicals it contains, known as yohimbine, increases fat mobilization and decreases fat reserves. No safe and effective dosage has been developed, as with most supplements.

These supplements are not explicitly tested and licensed by the FDA and are not reviewed by medical experts in a controlled sample. Claims are often founded on the hearsays, small numbers, or even exaggeration of unregulated individuals. For actual clinical trials, their arguments are almost all found to be unsubstantiated, sometimes the same as a placebo, often negative.

CHAPTER 4: DIET RECIPES FOR PCOS

Do not encourage a polycystic ovary syndrome (PCOS) condition to make you believe like you have lost control over your body. Ten million women worldwide suffer from hormonal and metabolic disorders, and symptoms – such as infertility, increase in weight, excess body hair, and androgen 'masculine' hormone production – are linked to insulin resistance. Although medicines such as Glucophage (metformin) and hormonal birth control are widely used for alleviation of the symptoms, your diet will help you feel your best. Healthy food is one thing you can do to take it back every day.

The right diet will help decrease PCOS symptoms by reducing inflammation and resistance to insulin. One thing is a warning. There's not one ideal PCOS diet, but it's clear that an anti-inflammatory diet focused on whole foods is the basis for your eating choices. That means you are free to eat in ways that will be nice to you while there are specific guidelines — focused on low-GI, fiber-rich products (leafy greens and avocados are two examples), grass-fed meats, organic poultry, nuts and seed and omega-3s (fatty fish, walnuts).

While you may be thinking of restriction with the term "diet" — especially if your doctor tells you to lose weight — this mustn't be the case. Focusing on taking care of yourself and practicing self-love techniques (good food is undoubtedly one) will help your body shift to a more relaxed position of health and healing.

1. How to create your platform to better manage PCOS

Start by creating real whole foods. Next, you can easily create nutritious food by concentrating on your plate. Recommends reserving half the plate for leafy greens and non-tactic vegetables. First, one-fifth of the program consists of starchy vegetables (examples of sweet potatoes), or gluten-free whole grains (e.g., quinoa). Lean protein is reserved for the last portion. Finally, add healthy fats (such as extra-virgin olive oil or nuts) to your food. Creating such a plate ensures you get the correct portion sizes. Therefore, you should be pleased with the fact that you will eventually stay away from pro-inflammatory foods like pure garbage and sugar.

2. The fatty acids, such as chia seeds, are historically praised as heart safe and anti-inflammatory in tuna, sardines, and vegetables. Focus on Foods with Omega-3 Fatty acids in one study with PCOS, and omega-three supplements reduced blood testosterone (a male hormone) for eight weeks relative to placebo. Besides, 47% of the omega-3 group repeated regular menstrual cycles compared with 23%. The researchers note that omega 3 helps to control luteinizing hormone levels, a testosterone secretion-stimulating hormone. Naturally, these women took supplements (3 grams of omega-3s daily). It is at least half a 3-ounce portion of salmon, so if you are not an ardent fish eater, you might find a substitute for the amount you need.

3. Eat a Bigger Breakfast to raise hormone levels. Another question is how the calories will be split all day long. Many people would save dinner as their most important meal of the day, but "eat a lavish breakfast, lunch like a princess and dinner as a wretch."

One research divided lean women with PCOS (their BMIs were approximately 24) into two groups; one ate breakfast with 980 calories (640 and 190 calories were lunch and dinner respectively), and the other ate a 190-calorie breakfast (640 and 980 respectively). Testosterone levels decreased by 50 percent after 90 days in the broad breakfast group and were more likely to ovulate while dinner groups did not shift. Eating earlier in the day possibly increased insulin sensitivity and reduced the amount of androgen, study authors conclude. It might not be possible to consume almost 1,000 calories at breakfast, but it might be worth trying to eat a bigger breakfast and a smaller dinner generally.

4. Select Glycemic Index (GI)

Foods low on the glycemic index (low GI) won't spike the blood glucose, and others are related to increased sensitivity to insulin. Yummy seeds like apples, berries, salads, kale, spinach, pumpkin seeds, cassava, and oats are recommended. Low-GI picks should usually pay dividends for your safety. In females without PCOS, higher-GI foods were associated with a higher waist and "poor" LDL cholesterol, and lower "healthy" HDL cholesterol. This is important because elevated levels of cholesterol are a significant factor in heart disease and are at higher risk for women with PCOS.

5. Stop Foods that tend to be Annoy

You all have foods that they do not handle well. Learn regarding your food intolerances or sensitivities (which, after you consume them, cause you gastrointestinal discomforts such as bloating, indigestion, and gas) and then prevent inflammation. If you have a gluten allergy, she says that you should start eating whole grains without gluten naturally (such as brown rice). She also suggests restricting milk and soy, but it is necessary to consult with your doctor to find out if these foods are the blame. Again, for everyone, there's no ideal PCOS diet! Often, by following a suppression diet in which you can eliminate all sources of these foods for three weeks, you can help decide whether you are intolerant to these foods, then add them at once and report all the symptoms. In this way, you can determine what your machine is troubling and what you can stop.

6. Lose weight if you need, and your PCOS symptoms can improve

One thing that is frequently clear in research is that weight-loss diets are good for alleviating PCOS problems. In 2013 a systematic analysis analyzed the best diet for PCOS in essence and concluded that weight loss improved symptoms (menstrual irregularities, insulin resistance, mood problems) regardless of the diet form. "We know that a small loss of weight helps with PCOS symptoms, but when you start to detoxify the body, the pressure is gone, she says. (After all, you may lose weight with an unhealthy diet because you consume fewer calories, but you don't feel right.) Focus on consuming foods rich in nutrients rather than worrying, whether it is small or high in carbohydrates, fat, or protein.

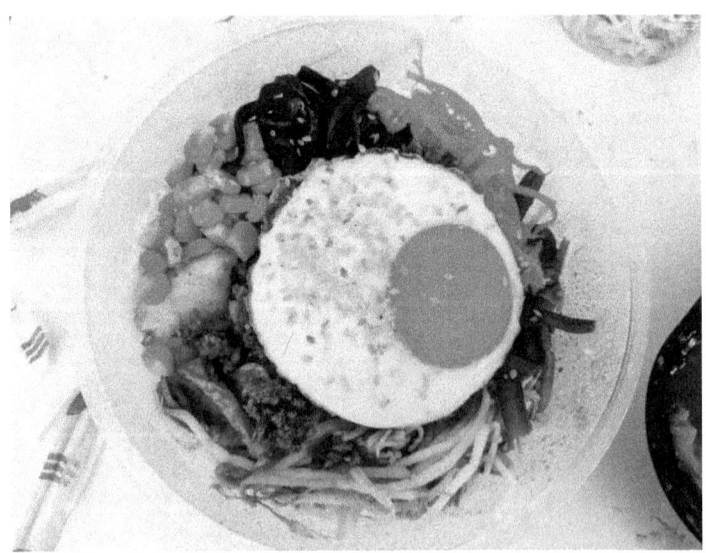

4.1 Breakfast

1. OVERNIGHT OATS

Ingredients:

- 1 cup of simple almond milk yogurt
- 1/3 cup uncooked oats
- 1/4 apple diced
- 10 grapes split in half (you may also use fresh berries)
- 6 walnuts
- 2 teaspoons of almond milk
- 3 drops of liquid stevia
- Cinnamon to fit

Directions:

Combine both ingredients the night before. Place in a glass jar that is sealed in a refrigerator. Note: If you consume milk, you will be able to substitute organic pure Greek yogurt for almond milk yogurt.

2. FAST AVOCADO TOAST

Ingredients:

- Single serving of pre-made guacamole, such as Solely Guacamole
- 2 or 3 eggs either hard-boiled and sliced or fried if you want
- 2 slices of tomato (optional)
- 2 slices of Ezekiel scattered grain bread, toasted

Directions:

Scatter the guacamole over the toast top with a sliced hard-boiled egg or scrambled eggs. Salt and chili pepper to compare. You should use sweet potato toast if you are allergic to gluten.

3. SCRAMBLED EGG & TOMATO SANDWICH

Ingredients:

- 4 slices of whole-grain bread
- 1 teaspoon of butter
- 2 cloves of garlic, finely chopped and peeled (optional)
- 2 teaspoons of dried parsley
- 1 cup of egg replacement (or four eggs), lightly beaten
- 2 big tomatoes, cored and finely chopped
- 1/4 teaspoon of salt

- 1/8 teaspoon of pepper
- 12 new basil plants, sliced or 1 1/2 teaspoons of dried basil

Directions:

Place butter in a medium-sized pan over low heat. Add garlic, parsley, and simmer for 2-3 minutes until butter melts. Attach the eggs and mix gently over low heat until fixed and cooked clean. Add salt and pepper to the mixture. Toast the bread lightly in the toaster. Arrange and split the egg mixture into four pieces of toasted bread. Cover each of them with basil leaves and scatter with cheese. Serve open-face sandwiches promptly, with a fork and a knife.

Requires four servings

4. PCOS FRIENDLY BREAD

Ingredients:

- 2 x cups whitened almond flour
- 2 x tablespoons coconut flour
- 1/4 x cup of golden flax flour
- 1/4 x cup of golden flax flour
- 1/4 x teaspoon of Celtic sea salt
- 1/2 x teaspoon of baking soda

- 5 x large eggs
- 1 tablespoon of apple cider vinegar

Directions:

Pulse almond flour, coconut flour, linseed, salt, and baking soda in a food processor. Pulse the eggs and the vinegar until combined. Transfer batter to 7.5 x 3.5 Magic Line Loaf Pan. Bake at 350 ° C for 30 minutes. Cool in the pan for 2 hours. Serve 8 Ingredients Need 40 Time (minutes)

5. PCOS FRIENDLY BACON ZUCCHINI LOAF

Ingredients :

- 1 cup of almond flour
- 3/4 cup of coconut flour
- 1/2 tsp. of salt
- 1 tsp. of baking soda
- 1 tsp. of nutritional yeast (optional)
- 1 tsp. of pepper
- 3 eggs
- 1/4 cup of coconut oil
- 3 strips of bacon, diced + 1 strip of top
- 1 cup of grated zucchini + a few slices of top

- a handful of fresh parsley, chopped Met Preheat oven to 360F/180C and grease loaf to tin

Directions:

In a container, combine all the dry ingredients. Combine all wet ingredients (excluding bacon, courgette, and parsley) in a separate pot. To dry the wet ingredients, blend well. Mix the bacon, the grated zucchini, and the parsley. Pour all of the batters in the loaf tin and decorate with the bacon strip and the zucchini slices. Bake for + -55 minutes or until the cake tester is clean.

6. LOW CARB KETO MUFFINS WITH BLACKBERRIES

The best recipe for LOW CARB MUFFINS! Such balanced muffins are packed with blackberries, free from butter, free from wheat, and free from sugar.

Ingredients

- 190 g Blackberries (fresh or frozen (or some other fruit)) Preheat the oven to 180 ° C/350 ° F.

Directions:

Fill up the muffin tray with 12 cups of muffin. Balance the blackberries with the starch of the coconut. Blend the dry ingredients in a large pot. Blend the wet ingredients in another big bowl. Mix the wet ingredients into the dry ones and blend them. It's not meant to be pourable, nor will it be too dense. It's intended to be spoon able. Attach the blackberries to the batter and blend properly. Place the muffin batter equally in 12 muffin cups. Then Put in oven to cook for 35 minutes. Test with a toothpick after 35 minutes to see whether the middle is either raw or not. The toothpick placed in the center is expected to come out clean. Now, Take the muffins out of the oven and allow them to cool off before eating. To freeze it, just cover it in a saran wrap or place it in a Ziploc container. To thaw the frozen muffins: move the frozen biscuits to the refrigerator and let them thaw for a few hours or place them on the counter and let them thaw for a few hours.

For sweetener substitutions, refer to the following:

- 1/2 cup (8 tbsp.) Surin Gold
- 6 tbsp. Lakanto Golden
- 1/2 cup (8 tbsp.)

So Nourished Monk Fruit Blend

- 1/2 cup (8 tbsp.) Swerve (not recommended as it leaves a considerable aftertaste)
- 1/2 cup (8 tbsp.) Erythritol + 1/4 tsp. stevia extract powder

- 1/2 cup (8 tbsp.) Erythritol + 1/4 tsp. monk fruit extract powder I choose the lemon juice for the flavor of the fruit.

Directions:

You should use sour cream instead of coconut milk. You can use olive oil, shortening, lard, butter, or ghee instead of coconut oil. You can use some other form of nut flour instead of almond flour. You can use any sort of berries or fruit you like instead of blackberries. Just remember to attach extra carbs to your nutritional facts. Make sure you use distilled coconut oil and not extra virgin coconut oil. The extra virgin smells so much like coconut, so it's going to spoil the flavor of the muffins! Make sure you use coconut cream and not coconut milk! Be sure you have muffin cups as the muffin batter likes to cling to the muffin pans even when oiled. Be sure that the coconut flour or blackberry muffin dough is not warm.

7. CHICKEN & APPLE BREAKFAST SAUSAGE WITH BAKED SWEET POTATO

Ingredients:

- 4 Applegate Naturals Chicken & Apple Breakfast Sausage Links

- 1 Sweet Potato
- 1/2 teaspoon Coconut Butter

Directions:

Bake Sweet Potato at a temperature of 400 ° F for 45 minutes. You should render your hair and making-up as it's frying or even microwave your potato for 8-10 minutes. Cook the sausage according to the directions of the maker. Cover the sweet potato with the butter of coconut and eat!

8. PALEO SPIRAL VEGETABLE TART

A crumbly gluten-free low-carb spiral vegetable pie with milk-free cashew cream. This makes two pies (8 slices each)

Ingredients:

- 2-4 eggplants (approximately 550 g)
- 4 zucchini/summer squash (about 600 g)
- 2 carrots (around 400 g)
- 2 tbsp. extra virgin olive oil
- 1/2 tsp. Himalayan salt Combine all the ingredients of the cashew cream in a food processor and pulse until the paste is smooth.

Directions:

In a large bowl, combine flour, salt, pepper, beef fat, and eggs. Blend with your hands or a spatula of silicone until a ball shapes the mixture. Separate in 2 since we've been making two pies. Put the dough on a sheet of paper and cover it with a fresh layer of paper. With a pin rolling slowly start to run it in a circular shape, 10-11 inches long, long enough to fill a 9 "glass pie plate. Remove the top piece of parchment paper and fold the dough carefully on the pie plate. To keep the pastry rolled up, press the pastry against the cake plate. Carefully remove the paper and fix any issues you may have. Repeat the second pie—Spread 1/2 of the cashew cream over the bottom of each cake.

Preheat the oven to 190C/375F oven. Peel the carrots and cut off all the vegetables from the stems. Slice all vegetables lengthwise with a mandolin slicer. Roll a small slice of zucchini into a tight ring and wrap a few more slices around. Place in the middle and start packing and rolling random slices of vegetables around the pie until you reach the crust. Carrots are the hardest to cover because they are less versatile than other vegetables. Dry an olive oil tablespoon and sprinkle over the entire cake with half the salt and pepper. Repeat the second pie cycle. Bake 40-45 minutes in the oven or until browning begins. Allow 10 minutes to cool before cutting.

This recipe makes two 9 "pies. Alternate between different colored vegetables to make a different colored pie.

9. MICROWAVE EGG AND VEGGIE BREAKFAST

Ingredient:

- 2 x eggs
- 1 x tbsp. Water
- 2 x tablespoons. Slender sliced baby spinach
- 2 x tbsp. Cut mushrooms
- Cut grape or cherry tomatoes
- 1/2 x cup strawberries, to serve

Directions:

The 8-oz coat. A ramekin or a custard cup with a cooking spray. Add the eggs, water, spinach, and mushrooms; beat until blended. MICROWAVE HIGH 30 seconds; stir. Microwave until the egg is almost fixed, 30 to 45 seconds longer. Top with some tomatoes. Serve on the side with a 1/2 cup of strawberries.

This food is a good source of niacin, foliate, vitamin B12, pantothenic acid, iron, phosphorous, potassium, copper and manganese, and an excellent source of protein, vitamin A, vitamin C, vitamin K, riboflavin and selenium. It's also MILDLY anti-inflammatory.

Ingredients:

- 1 x tbsp. Olive oil
- 2 x large zucchini (courgette), chopped into small pieces
- 7 oz. (200 g) pack of cherry tomatoes, halved
- 1 x clove of garlic, crushed
- 4 x eggs
- few leaves of basil, to serve

Direction:

In a nonstick casserole, heat the oil and add the corvettes. Fry for 5 minutes, continually stirring until cooked, add the tomatoes and garlic, then simmer for a few more minutes. Stir in a little spice, then put the mixture into two holes and break the eggs. Cover the cup with a lid or foil sheet and cook for 2 to 3 minutes to get your eggs cooked. Layover several leaves of basil, and drink.

This diet is a good source of calcium, vitamin C, vitamin K, riboflavin, potassium, manganese and selenium, and an excellent source of vitamin A. It is slightly anti-inflammatory too.

10. INSTANT FLAX MEAL ALMOND BUTTER HOT CEREAL

Ingredients:

- 1/4 cup linseed meal (ground linseed)
- 1/2 cup boiling water
- 1 x tbsp. Almond butter
- 1/4 tsp. Cinnamon
- 1/2 grapefruit

Directions:

Pour boiling water over the linseed meal and stir well. Stir in cinnamon and almond butter. Let it thicken for 1 to 2 minutes. Serve with a half grapefruit.

4.2 Lunch

1. MISO EGGPLANT RECIPE MISO EGGPLANT

Ingredients:

- 1 big eggplant
- 1 tablespoon of vegetable/canola oil

- 1 tablespoon of white miso paste
- 1 tablespoon of mirin
- sesame seed

Directions:

Cut the eggplants in half with a sharp knife and split them in a cress-cross fashion, make sure you don't break through the flesh. Heat oil in a nonstick pan and apply the cut side of the eggplant. Cook for a few minutes until dark, then switch over, use two tablespoons of water and cover with a cap. Cook 4-5 minutes. Mix the miso paste, mirin, and oil in a tiny bowl and mix well to smooth out any lumps. Place the eggplant on the foil-lime tray and spoon the miso mixture to make sure it covers the gaps. Place the mixture under a hot grill and cook until it bubbles. Sprinkle with sesame seeds, toast, and drink while it's soft.

2. VEGETABLE LENTIL SOUP

Ingredients:

- 2 medium carrots
- 2 medium celery sticks
- 1 medium onion
- 4 small red potatoes
- 1 garlic clove
- 2 teaspoons of oil (olive, canola or vegetable)
- 1 cup of dried lentils
- 1 little head of escarole (about 1 pound)
- 2 (14 1/2 ounce) tins of chicken broth (low-sodium or regular)
- 1 (14 1/2 to 16 ounce) can Italian stewed tomatoes
- 3 cups of water

Directions:

Dice broccoli, celery, and onion; split the potatoes into 1/2 inch pieces; thin the garlic. Heat oil over medium-high heat in a five-quarters Dutch oven or big, heavy pot; add celery, carrots, and onions and cook mild, stirring periodically. Attach the garlic and cook, stirring, until the garlic starts to glow. Mix in the stewed tomatoes with their milk, dried lentils, chicken broth, potatoes and 3 cups of water; mix with a spoon to remove the vegetables. Take to a boil and raising the heat to be small. Cover and boil until the lentils are soft for around 50 minutes. Break the escarole as the soup is simmering. Just before eating, add the escarole to the soup and simmer, stirring regularly, until the escarole wilts. Makes five servings of Tip: Eat this meal with a whole-grain roll or a bread piece.

3. ROASTED BUFFALO CHICKPEA SALAD

Ingredients:

- 2 tablespoons of white vinegar, divided
- 1/2 teaspoon of cayenne pepper, or according to taste
- 1/4 teaspoon of salt plus a pinch, divided
- 1 (15 ounces) can't add chickpeas, rinsed
- 1 tablespoon of hot sauce, such as Frank's Red-hot
- 2 tablespoons of chickpeas

Directions:

In a large bowl, combine one tablespoon of vinegar, cayenne, and 1/4 teaspoon of salt. Dry the chickpeas very thoroughly, then toss with the mixture of vinegar. Spread it on a rimmed baking sheet. Roast the chickpeas, stirring twice, until browned and crispy, for 30 to 35 minutes. Transfer to a bowl small in size and mix in a hot sauce. In a large bowl, whisk oil, garlic powder, and the remaining one tablespoon of vinegar and a pinch of salt. Add the lettuce, carrots, celery, and chickpeas. Toss to combine it. Divide between 4 bowls and top with blue cheese. The chickpeas remain crisp at room temperature for 2 to 4 hours; if stored longer, return to 400 degrees F for 5 to 10 minutes.

4. COAL MINER'S SPAGHETTI

Easy and quick enough for a week's night meal, this spaghetti squash recipe warmed and fill us up. You're going to want to continue cooking squash ahead of time.

Ingredients:

- 1 big spaghetti squash, fried and twisted
- 2 teaspoons of olive oil
- 1/2 cup white wine (or regular chicken broth)
- 1/4 boiling water
- 8 oz. Prosciutto, minced
- 4 cloves of garlic, minced
- 1/2 tsp. of red pepper flakes (crushed)
- 2 egg yolks
- a pinch of parsley
- salt and pepper to taste

Directions:

Simply cut it in half and bake at 350 for 45 minutes. When it's cold, use a spoon to gut out the seeds. Then use a fork to curl the edges of the squash. This just seems like the pasta! In a full pan warmed to hot, sautéed. Attach the remaining olive oil, garlic, and crushed red pepper flakes and sauté for 2 minutes. Attach the wine to the pan and that too half, about 1 minute. In a separate pot, pound the egg yolks together and stir in hot water while whisking vigorously. Add spaghetti squash, egg mixture, parsley, salt, and pepper and stir for 2 minutes. Garnish it and protect it.

5. HAM AND CHEESE ROLL-UPS

Ingredients:

- 2 lettuce or four small leaves, washed
- 2 pieces of thin, lean ham
- 4 small pieces of hard cheese, sliced into thin strips (I used Jarlsberg)

Directions:

Lay the leaf down and then roll it up with ham and cheese strips.

6. BRAISED CELERY

Ingredients:

- 4 long celery stalks, cleaned and cut diagonally, leaves removed
- 1 cup of chicken stock or one cube of Massel dissolved in hot water
- 1 large clove of garlic minced
- Black pepper

Directions:

Cut the celery on diagonal 2 in 1 cm bits. In a small pan, put the stock to a boil. Add some celery and garlic. Cover the pan and reduce the heat to simmer for 5-10 minutes, depending on how soft it is. Stretch the liquid and remove it. Serve with a healthy twist of black pepper.

7. BUTTERNUT AND LENTIL SOUP

Ingredients:

- 1 x medium Onion (Chopped)
- 2 x cloves Garlic (Minced)
- 2 x cups Butternut (Peeled and Diced)
- 1 x cup Carrot (Peeled and Sliced)

- 6 x cups Vegetable stock
- Scatter Mixed Herbs
- 1 x tablespoon Olive Oil
- 1 cup Red Lentils

Directions:

Prepare the butternut, carrot, and onion by peeling and slicing. Heat the olive oil gently and cook the carrots, onions, and garlic until the onions are tender. Add 4 cups of vegetable storage, milk, lentils, spices, and cayenne chili pepper. Simmer for 30-45 minutes until batter is smooth. Mix the broth until it's creamy. Add more stock before the target quality is achieved. Continue mixing to ensure that the soup is mixed correctly and condensed.

8. KETO PALEO BONE BROTH

Ingredients:

- 1 Dutch Oven Roasted Chicken with its LEFTOVERS

Directions:

When your roast chicken is baked, take it out of the Dutch oven and leave with some soft vegetable scraps and some chicken juice. Don't give it away. We're going to use this to create the Delicious bone broth. After you've cut all the meat out of the chicken carcass, put all the bones back in the Dutch oven over the vegetables. Apply water to the Dutch oven before the bones are sealed. I just added around 2L. Cover the lid and put the Dutch oven back in the furnace of 190C/375F for 3 hours. Three hours is outstanding for a 1 kg bird. If you have used 2 kg of chicken, cook it for 4 hours. After 3 hours in the oven, take it out of the oven. Remove significant bits (bones and vegetables) with a pair of tongues and strains. Take the Dutch oven and drain it through the filter. Remove the plants and the bones and place them in the cheesecloth. You want to suck as much juice out of these as you can! All the flavor is in the vegetables, so you're going to squeeze fast! * You might want to let the broth cool down first because it's going to be hot pipes! * 6.-6. After you are done draining all the liquid from the bones and vegetables, you should discard it. Then you're left with a beautiful homemade bone broth! Hold whatever you want to drink in a refrigerator jar this week. You can freeze the leftover soup in some ice cubes or some silicone muffin cups for later use.

9. CHICKEN AND BLACK BEAN BURRITOS

4 Servings Calories per serving: 360 calories

When you haven't wanted to eat a burrito before, you haven't eaten yet! Mexican food is an enjoyable way to spice up your meal. It's super simple to produce, and depending on the products you choose, it can also be super safe! We're going to use chicken and vegetables in this recipe, and you're going to believe this one is safe. Let's think about black beans, however. Who creates burrito-worthy black beans? Black beans or turtle beans are known as legumes. Like other legumes — peanuts, peas, and lentils — these beans are especially rich in fiber. One cup of cooked black beans produces 15 grams of fiber. Research has shown that eating a high-fiber diet will help raise blood sugar rates.

Ingredients and directions:

- 1 avocado, crushed
- 4 big whole-wheat tortillas
- 1/2 jar of salsa
- 2 cups of cooked chicken breast, sliced
- 1 cup of dried non-salted black beans, rinsed and drained

- 6 tablespoons of reduced-fat shredded cheddar cheese
- 1 cup of shredded lettuce
- 1 cup of diced tomatoes
- Pack the tortilla in the burrito and dive deep!

10. SUSHI ROLLS

Ingredients:

- 100 g of smoked salmon, cut into small pieces
- 1/2 avocado, thinly sliced
- Nora sheets
- 2 shallots, cut into long slices
- Wasabi
- Soy sauce for dipping

Directions:

Cut the sheets of nor into large squares. Add the smoked salmon, the sliced avocado, and the shallots diagonally to the non-shiny side. Roll up in a cone. Seal the end of it with a little water to make it stick. Serve with wasabi and soya sauce for dipping.

11. AVOCADO AND GRILLED SALMON

Salad 4 Servings

Calories per serving: 320 calories

This recipe is full of fat — well, the kind of fat you'd want to place in your mouth and your stomach since it's "good" fat! We recognize that salmon is one of the fatty fish that is filled with heart-healthy omega-3 fatty acids. As for avocado, it turns out that there is a much higher explanation why it exists — apart from, you know, offering us mouth-watering guacamoles! Avocados are filled with monounsaturated fatty acids (MUFAs) — another source of healthy fat — known to boost the right level of cholesterol. Such fatty acids can also reduce the rates of bad cholesterol and triglycerides. Healthy fats like salmon and avocado will help reduce the likelihood of heart failure and stroke, which are significant health issues for people with diabetes.

Ingredients

- 4 4-oz frozen salmon fillets, roasted
- 1 tablespoon of olive oil
- 1 tablespoon of no-salt grilled seasoning
- 4 cups of roman lettuce
- 1/2 cup of red onion (thinly sliced)
- 1 cup of cucumber

- 1 cup of mature avocado, trimmed, trimmed and cut

Dressing:

- 1/4 cup of lime juice
- 1 tablespoon of lime

Directions:

Dry the dipped salmon fillets with a paper towel and then sprayed the olive oil on each leg. Season the filets with the no-salt grill seasoning. Grill the fillets of salmon for between 4-5 minutes on either side or until cooked clean. Place it back. Complete Romaine lettuce with sliced tomato, sliced cucumber, fried salmon filet, and avocado slices. Shake together the lime juice, the olive oil, the Dijon mustard, the stevia, the salt, and the pepper and drizzle over the dish.

12. MEDITERRANEAN CAULIFLOWER PIZZA

In this healthy, gluten-free 'pizza' cauliflower recipe, shredded cauliflower is mixed with mozzarella and oregano to make a flour-free crust that echoes the flavor of a traditional pizza. Meyer's orange, olive, and sun-dried tomato tops add an elegant Mediterranean flavor but try more common pizza toppings such as marinara and mushroom — even pepperoni.

Ingredients:

- 1 medium head cauliflower (approximately 2 pounds), trimmed and broken into small flowers
- 1 tablespoon plus one teaspoon of extra virgin olive oil, divided
- 1/4 teaspoon of salt
- 2 Meyer lemons or one large standard lemon
- 6 sun-dried oil-packed tomatoes, washed, rusted
- 1/3 cup green or black, sliced and pitted
- 1 large egg, slightly b A pizza pot or a rimless parchment paper bakery.

Directions:

In a food processor, put cauliflower and pulse until it is reduced to rice crumbs. Switch to a large nonstick pot and add one cubic cubicle of oil and salt. Heat at medium-high, stir regularly until the coolant gradually starts to soften (but don't let it brown) for 8 to 10 minutes. Switch to a full bowl for a minimum of 10 minutes to cool. Remove the skin and white pit from the lemon(s) with a sharp knife and discard it. Cut the membrane segments over a small bowl and drop them into the pot (remove the seeds). Delete the pieces of the juice (save for further use). In the lemon parts, add tomatoes and olives; mix to combine. In the chopped cauliflower, add the potato, cheese, and oregano; mix well. Spread the mixture onto the bakery board, making a diameter of 10 inches. Drizzle over the top the remainder of one teaspoon of oil. Drizzle the remaining one teaspoon of oil over the top. Bake the pizza until the top is brown, 10 to 14 minutes. Spread the lemon-olive mixture over the top, season with pepper, and continue to cook until well browned for 8 to 14 minutes. Stretch the basil over the top. Cut the wedges and serve.

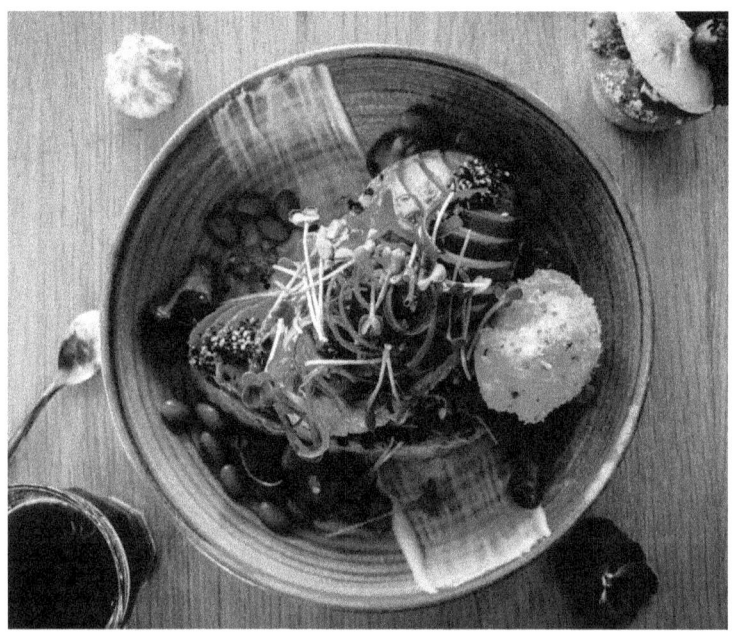

4.3 Dinner

1. MISO GRILLED VEGETABLES

Ingredients:

- 2 tablespoons of white miso paste
- 1 tablespoon of water
- 3 tablespoons of vegetable oil
- 2 zucchini, sliced diagonally z
- 1 large red pepper, cut into large pieces
- Optional:
- 1 small eggplant, sliced lengthwise
- 1 small red onion, cut into wedges
- 1 green pepper, cut into large pieces

Directions:

In a bowl, combine miso paste with water and whisk until smooth. Gradually add the oil to the thin stream until it emulsifies. Add the sliced vegetables and mix well to coat all the surfaces. Grill on the barbecue until cooked.

2. BROCCOLI, CHICKPEA & POMEGRANATE SALAD

Simple measures give this broccoli salad a more complex taste: The onion soaks its crunch, and cumin toast enhances the aroma. Serve with chicken, pork, or fish grilled.

Ingredients:

- 1/4 cup thinly sliced red onion
- 1/2 teaspoon ground cumin
- 1/3 cup whole-milk plain yogurt
- 2 tablespoons tahini
- 2 tablespoons extra virgin olive oil
- 1 tablespoon lemon juice
- 3/4 teaspoon salt, divided
- 1/2 teaspoon ground pepper
- 4 cups of broccoli flowers (about 8 ounces)

Directions:

(15 ounces) can low-sodium chickpeas, rinsed Well, drain well. Meanwhile, toast the cumin over medium heat in a small dry skillet, blend until sparkling, for 1 to 2 minutes. Transfer to a deep tub. Transfer. Attach yogurt, tahini, olive oil, lemon juice, 1/2 salt, and pepper powder, whisk to smooth. Add broccoli, chickpeas, grenade seeds, onion, and toss. Let stand 10 minutes. Let stand. Apply 1/4 of a teaspoon of salt and whisk again. Refrigerate for up to 1 day.

3. MARMALADE CHICKEN WITH WILD RICE AND SAUTEED SPINACH

Ingredients:

- 1/2 x cup reduced-sodium chicken broth
- 1 x tablespoon red-wine vinegar
- 1 x tablespoon orange marmalade
- 1/2 x teaspoon Dijon mustard
- 1/2 x teaspoon cornstarch
- 8 oz. (227 g) x chicken tender
- 1/4 x teaspoon kosher salt
- 1/8 x teaspoon freshly ground pepper
- 1 x tablespoon extra-virgin olive oil, divided
- 1 x large shallot, minced
- 1/2 x teaspoon freshly ground pepper

Directions:

In a small cup, whisk, sugar, marmalade, mustard, and cornstarch. Sprinkle with salt and pepper over the chicken. Heat 2 teaspoons of oil in a large saucepan over medium-high heat. Attach the chicken and cook until golden, around 2 minutes per hand. Switch to the plate and cover with foil to keep dry. Attach the remaining one teaspoon of oil and shallot to the pan and cook until crispy, frequently stirring, for about 30 seconds. Whisk the mixture and add it to the oven. Reduce heat to keep simmering; cook until sauce is gently reduced and thickened for 30 seconds to 2 minutes. Add the chicken, go back to simmering. Cook, turning once until chicken is heated for around 1 minute. Remove from oil, add in the orange peel. While the chicken is simmering, sauté the spinach in a small amount of olive oil. Serve with sautéed spinach and wild rice

4. ALL-GRAIN SUSHI RICE

While typical white sushi rice, this brown sushi rice base is combined with other lentils and grains. Regular vinegar and sugar seasoning are omitted in this whole-grain brown sushi rice recipe so that the natural taste of the whole grain shines through. Any lentils work — French green lentils are best shaped.

Ingredients:

- 1 1/4 cups of short grain brown rice
- 1/4 cup wild rice
- 1/4 cup lentils
- 1/4 cup quinoa

- 3 tablespoons ground linseed
- 4 cups warm water

Directions:

Mix brown rice, wild rice, lentils, quinoa, and linseed in a large saucepan; add water. Enable to stand at room temperature for at least 30 minutes and hydrate the grain for up to 4 hours. Place a small lid on the pot and bring to a boil. Reduce to very moderate, cook until almost the entire liquid evaporates for 35 to 40 minutes. Take off the heat and leave it covered for 30 minutes. Uncover it and get a little chilly for about 1 hour. Cover and cook for up to 3 days; carry to room temperature before making sushi.

Look for ground flaxseed (flax meal) in supermarkets or natural food stores or grind whole flaxseed in a clean coffee blender just before using it—place in the refrigerator or freezer.

5. SPAGHETTI SQUASH LASAGNA WITH BROCCOLINI

In this low-carb spaghetti squash lasagna recipe, garlic broccoli, spaghetti squash, and cheese are mixed to make the most of the classic casserole. This is baked right in the squash shells for an excellent show. Serve with a large Caesar salad and some hot and crusty whole-grain bread.

Ingredients:

- 1 1/2 to 3-pound spaghetti squash, halved in length and seeded
- 1 tablespoon extra-virgin olive oil
- 1 bunch of broccoli, chopped
- 4 cloves of garlic, minced
- 1/4 teaspoon of crushed red pepper (optional)
- 2 tablespoons of water
- 1 cup of shredded mozzarella cheese

Directions:

Put the cut-side squash in a microwave-safe dish; attach two tablespoons of water. Microwave, exposed, on Fast, until the flesh is soft, perhaps ten minutes. (Alternatively, put the squash cut-side down on a rimmed baking sheet. Bake in 400 degrees F oven until the squash is soft, for 40 to 50 minutes.)

In the meantime, heat oil in a big skillet over medium heat. Attach broccoli, garlic, and red pepper (if used); cook, constantly stirring, for 2 minutes. Remove the water and cook, stirring until the broccoli is soft, 3 to 5 more minutes. Switch to a deep tub. Using a fork to push the shell squash into the pot. Place the shells in a broiler-safe pan or on a baking sheet. Stir in the squash mixture 3/4 cup mozzarella, two teaspoons Parmesan, Italian seasoning, salt, and pepper. Divide between the shells; finish with the remaining 1/4 cup of mozzarella and two teaspoons of parmesan. Bake on the bottom rack for almost 10 minutes. Switch to the top shelf, turn the appliance to the peak and broil, watch closely before the cheese begins to brown for around 2 minutes. To save your time and keep your baking sheet new, line it with a coat of foil until you bake.

6. SWEDISH MEATBALLS WITH GARLIC BRUSSELS & ZUCCHINI

Ingredients:

- 2 tsp. olive oil
- 1 small onion, minced
- 2 cloves garlic, minced
- 1/4 cup rosemary, chopped

- 1 lb. 93 percent lean beef (see vegan if possible, no additional hormones)
- 1 egg
- salt and pepper to taste
- 2 cups natural beef stock

Directions:

In a deep sauté pan, heat medium oil and add onions and garlic until the onions are trance. Attach the romaine and cook until tender. Keep it fresh for a few minutes. Mix beef, potato, onion mixture, and salt and pepper in a full pot. Mix well and shape balls with your hands, around 1/8 cup each. Test for 1/4 cup and half. Remove beef stock and put it to a boil. Reduce and slowly add the meatballs to the broth. Cover and simmer for about 20 minutes.

For Brussels and Zucchini

Ingredients:

- 2 teaspoons of olive oil
- 5 oz. Brussels, trimmed and cut thin
- 1 small zucchini, sliced and halved
- 3 cloves of garlic, minced

Directions:

Heat oil in a saucepan over less heat. Add the garlic and sauté for 3-4 minutes. Attach the sprouts and the zucchini. Cook until finely soft, stirring, about 5-6 minutes. Reduce heat and cook for 3-4 more minutes. Let it cool and serve.

7. ONE PAN SALMON

ONE PAN Salmon is a perfect PCOS friendly dinner. It's a decent source of essential Omega 3 fatty acids. And we learn that Omega 3 allows reducing testosterone rates and inflammation of the rash. If you're purchasing fish, consider getting wild Alaskan fish or some other wild salmon that is far richer in Omega 3 than farmed salmon.

Ingredients:

- 1 lb./400 g of new potatoes, halved if big
- 2 tbsp. of olive oil
- 8 asparagus spears, trimmed and halved
- 2 handfuls of cherry tomatoes
- 1 tbsp. of balsamic vinegar
- 2 filets of salmon, roughly 140g/5 oz. each
- a handful of basil leaves

Directions:

Heat oven to 430F/220C. Here is a Tip the potatoes and 1 tbsp. of olive oil in an ovenproof dish, then fry the potatoes for 20 minutes until crispy. Toss the asparagus in with the carrots, and move to the oven for 15 minutes. Throw tomatoes and vinegar into the cherry tomatoes, nest salmon between the vegetables. Drizzle the remaining oil and return to the oven for the last ten to fifteen minutes before the salmon is fried. Scatter over the basil leaves and eat from the bowl, all scooped.

8. MISO GRILLED VEGETABLES

Ingredients:

- 2 tablespoons of white miso paste
- 1 tablespoon of water
- 3 tablespoons of vegetable oil
- 2 zucchini, sliced diagonally
- 1 large red pepper, cut into large pieces
- Optional:
- 1 small eggplant, sliced lengthwise
- 1 small red onion, cut into wedges
- 1 green pepper, cut into large pieces

Directions:

In a bowl, combine miso paste with water and whisk until smooth. Gradually add the oil to the thin stream until it emulsifies. Add the sliced vegetables and mix well to coat all the surfaces. Grill on the barbecue until cooked.

9. BALSAMIC GLAZED SALMON

We also know that losing excess pounds because you're overweight and adding muscle mass — because we don't want to add body fat while we're striving to raise "weight " — because you're underweight is beneficial for your safety. And while you're attempting to control insulin resistance, preserving your "ideal" body weight is highly critical. Yeah, how are you going to feed your way through losing weight? Poultry and fish are your most reliable choice. For example, they are smaller in calories relative to pork and beef. Salmon, the critical ingredient in this recipe, is one of the healthiest fish out there. Oozing with omega-3 fatty acids — a healthy form of fat — may help reduce the risk of heart disease and lower blood pressure.

Ingredients:

- 1/2 cup balsamic vinegar
- 2 teaspoons Dijon mustard
- 2 teaspoons of honey

- 2 4-oz salmon fillets
- 1/2 green onion, sliced

Directions:

Preheat oven to 400 degrees Fahrenheit. In a small saucepan, mix vinegar, Dijon mustard, and honey and bring to a boil over medium heat. Simmer for almost ten minutes or until the consistency is deep. Using part of the balsamic glaze in salmon fillets. Cook the filets of glazed salmon for 10-14 minutes. Remove the cooked salmon from the oven. Pour over the remaining glaze. Finish with green onion and serve wet.

10. CAULIFLOWER FRIED "RICE"

A delicious low-carb alternative to regular white rice!

Ingredients:

- 1 cauliflower (medium)
- 1/4 onion
- 2 slices ham
- 2 stems green onions
- 1 tbsp. coconut amines
- 2 tbsp. sesame oil
- 1 tsp. Himalayan salt

- 1 tsp. coconut amines

- 2 eggs

- 1 tsp. black pepper

Directions:

Divide the blooms from the cauliflower and put them in a food processor. Chop until the florets are like "rice grains." Consider onions and ham. Slice green onions. Slice them. Heat some sesame oil in a wok. Attach the onions and flower cauliflower. Start to fry until the cauliflower and the onions become translucent. Attach the green onions and ham. Cook for another two minutes. Fill in soy, salt and pepper, and dash powder. Mix well and cook for 2 minutes. Move the fried rice to the pan side and scatter the eggs around the plate. Start scrambling them, start climbing them. When tossed and wholly cooked, combine the rice and the eggs in the squad. Serve hot for another minute.

Dashy powder typically does not contain gluten. It's a Japanese powdered fish broth used to sample dishes. If you're not going to use it, just turn it to chicken or beef cubes.

11. KETO GLUTEN-FREE PIGS IN A SHEET

These low carb pigs in a layer are made of coconut flour, almond flour, and phylum husk powder. They're milk-free and don't use the fathead dough!

Ingredients:

- Eggs
- Boiling water
- Psyllium
- Coconut Flour
- Pork
- Bagel seasoning , Rolling Pin
- Large mixing bowl

The oven should be preheated to 180 ° C or 350 ° F temperature

Direction:

Add the dry ingredients in a large bowl and mix well with a whisk. Add the three eggs to the pan and mix well with the spatula. The dough will be a little difficult to blend, so use muscle! In 4 steps, pour in the boiling water and combine it with each pour. You should note that the coconut flour and the phylum absorb water when it is poured in. Mix the spatula dough until all the water is added. Knead the flour with your hands until there is a large disk. Divide the money into twelve equal balls. On top of the table, put a sheet of paper, place one shot in the middle, and cover with another piece of paper parchment. Push the ball to flatten it a bit, and then roll it out with a rolling pin about 15cm/6 "long and tens/4" wide (more than your sausage size). Place the sausage on the rolled dough and roll it in a roll. The sausage is to be covered entirely, but the tip and the end are to be seen. Repeat with the remaining dough and sausage. Transfer the pigs to the baking tray in a blanket. In a small bowl, combine one egg and 1 tbsp. of water. This is the washing of the egg. Brush it in a sheet on top of all the pigs. Sprinkle all but the bagel seasoning on top of it. Place in the oven and cook it for 25-30 minutes. The dough is softer for 25 minutes and crisper for 30 minutes. Take your favorite low carb dip sauces out of the oven!

- This recipe will NOT work without the power of the phylum husk.

- Make sure you use phylum husk powder and not whole shells. If you only have full tanks, make sure you grind them in a coffee grinder to turn them into a powder before use.

- They can be stuffed with some sort of sausage, ground beef, cheese, or vegetables. You are not limited to sausages.

- Be sure that the dough is rolled out between two pieces of parchment paper or that the mixture sticks to your roller pin or table.

- Make sure you use hot water and do not use warm water. The phylum is best activated by boiling water.

- You can use any form of seasoning you want instead of bagel seasoning.

12. ANTS ON LO

Ingredients:

- 1 teaspoon of peanut butter or soy nut butter
- 1 stalk celery
- Raisins

Directions:

Clean and cut the ends of the celery. Place the peanut butter or the soy nut butter on each celery block. Cover with a pair of raisins.

13. CHICKEN & ZUCCHINI IN WHITE WINE SAUCE

Quick and fast, this recipe is perfect for a simple week night's dinner. Any other veggie could substitute the zucchini. Butter makes this ideal, so don't skimp it, just use it! No leftovers from this one; double the recipe if you have babies.

Ingredients:

- 8 chicken tenderloins (more for larger families)
- 1 tbsp. light butter
- 2 tbsp. olive oil
- 3 tbsp. minced garlic
- 12 oz. sliced zucchini
- 1/4 cup white wine
- 1/3 cup low sodium chicken broth (may use fat-free, too)
- 1-2 tbsp. corn starch
- salt and pepper to taste
- 1/4 cup fresh parsley, chopped

Directions:

Heat ski meat Add 1/2 tbsp. of butter and olive oil when it is cold. Add salt and pepper to chicken and put it in a bowl. Cook about 7-8 minutes on each side until chicken is not rose anymore. Hold it moist and set aside in a different container. Apply 1/2 tbsp. of butter, olive oil, and garlic to the same pan. Attach the zucchini, salt, and pepper and roast for 5 minutes or until golden. Incorporate any rice, chicken broth, parsley, and cornstarch. Extract some pieces from the oven. Bring the heat up to the boil and reduce to minimum, cover and simmer for about 5 minutes until the liquid has thickened. Cover the chicken with the sauce and eat.

14. SHIRATAKI NOODLES AND INSULIN RESISTANCE

If diagnosed with insulin resistance, use shirataki noodles as a supplement for rice, noodles, and pasta. Shirataki Noodles Shirataki noodles are long, transparent noodles produced from konjac yam, a tuber containing glucomannan, which is a water-soluble dietary fiber known to extend when eaten. The original composition is filtered water, konjac rice, calcium hydroxide (a preservative reported to have no harmful effects). You may get them in fettuccine form, angel hair, and pasta, which is mainly thin noodles sliced into "bean" sizes. You may have learned of them as the Miracle Noodles or the Slender company.

Directions:

They arrive in a box floating in a liquid that tastes so fishy that you may be tempted to throw them away. Don't do it. Open the package over the toilet, place it in a colander and rinse it under hot water for 1-2 minutes. Place the filter in a full bowl and pour boiling water over it for 1-2 minutes. Strain, guy. They're good to go now. They've been in the refrigerator for no longer than two days.

Benefits of Shirataki Noodles

They can be a replacement for traditional pasta, rice, and noodles. In certain instances, they seem like the real deal when you only need some homemade stir-fry rice. There's minimal glucose or no food, small calories to no calories, and there's little remorse consuming them. When paired with the correct ingredients, they do not taste that bad.

Disadvantages of Shirataki Noodles

They have gastro-effects varying from flatulence, mild cramps, nausea, constipation, to all of the above. They can induce intestinal blockage. They're not supplying the body with much nutrients, just bulk and a sense of fullness, so you're going to be starving right after. Shirataki Noodles and Insulin Resistance or Shirataki noodles operate well by swallowing the sauce or by utilizing intense tastes in the cooking process. Don't eat the entire package at mealtime. Half a serving is appropriate, so bear in mind the side effects. Don't give them a diet or a fast way to lose weight. They've got too little calories. You may feel full right after you eat them, but soon you'll feel hungry. Consult with the doctor until they are used. After all, they are refined foods.

15. CAULIFLOWER AND SPINACH MASH

Ingredients:

- 1/4 x Teaspoon Garlic Powder
- 1/4 x Teaspoon Onion Powder
- 1 x Tablespoon Butter (optional)
- Salt and Pepper to taste

Directions:

Cut the flower head into the flowers and boil for 15 minutes or until soft when the fork is speared. Puree the cauliflower with a handheld blender. Add the spinach and proceed to blend until it is smooth. Add the remaining ingredients to make sure the mash is well blended and smooth.

16. SWEET ONION FRITTATA WITH HAM

4 Serving Calories per meal: 110 calories

Eggs, guy! A ton of people are nuts about eggs not just because they're safe, but also because they're easy to produce! There are several ways to cook and eat the eggs — sunny-side-up, frittata, omelet, fried, and you name it! Egg dishes are packed, particularly if you have fiber-rich vegetables in your recipe. Although the amount of cholesterol is what affects certain men. Eggs are rich in dietary cholesterol, providing more than two-thirds of the regular minimum cholesterol intake. And, in egg dishes that use, well, a lot of eggs — like this recipe — using egg replacements may be a smart option. Don't worry, as egg replacements are always good! Vitamins and minerals such as magnesium, foliate, thiamin, riboflavin, copper, vitamins A, C, B6, and B12 are introduced to account for the lack of yolk elimination.

Ingredients:

- 1 cup Texas Sweet Onion or Vidalia, thinly sliced
- 1 1/2 cup egg replacement
- 4 oz. of extra lean, low-sodium ham slices.
- 1/2 cup cooked, low-fat cheddar cheese

Directions:

Put a small nonstick skillet on medium-high heat until heated and then cover with cooking spray. Cook the ham for around 2-3 minutes or until it is softly gray. Remove and set aside from the skillet. Paint the saucepan with the cooking water. Cook the onion for around 4 minutes or until white. Remove the ham and cook for another minute, enabling the flavors to mix. Pour the egg mixture uniformly, cover, and simmer for around 8 minutes or until puffy and set. Delete the flame from the skillet. Sprinkle the cheese on top, cover, and leave stand for about 3 minutes before the cheese is melted.

4.4 Sweets

1. SUGAR-FREE NUTELLA

This fantastic chocolate hazelnut spread is the perfect sugar-free substitute you'll ever seek!

Prep Time 20 minutes Cook Time 15 minutes Total Time 35 minutes

Ingredients:

- 1 tbsp. of distilled coconut oil
- 4 tbsp. of chocolate powder

- 5 tbsp. of powdered erythritol and (1-1.5 tsp.) of stevia for paleo
- 400 g (14.11 oz.) of hazelnuts (about 2.5 cups)

Directions:

Attach the hazelnuts to the oven tray and roast at 160C/320F temperature. Bake for 15-20 minutes, after 10 minutes, then every so often to make sure they haven't burnt. Bring the pan out of the oven and clean the nuts together with a towel or an oven glove to remove their shells. Not all nut shells will break off, so that's all right. Only seek to extract as much crust as you can! Attach the hazelnuts to the healthy food processor and pulse for a minute before the flour. Attach the coconut oil to the food processor and steam for 8-10 minutes. Scrap the surfaces from time to time. The faster you cook it (and the better the food processor), the cleaner the Nutella becomes. I like mine very smooth and runny, and I've been processing it for about 10 minutes. Attach the cocoa powder and the erythritol to the food processor and cycle for another 2 minutes. It's all finished and ready to serve! Place in a jar or Tupperware refrigerator. It's expected to last 3-4 weeks.

2. CHOCOLATE CHEESECAKE PUMPKIN SQUARES

Carbs come from graham crackers, but they are made of whole grain and have healthy protein and fiber in them and relatively low in sugar. Some carbohydrates come from the devil himself, man! Yeah, pure sugar in this one, guys. We often want to make it with a full cup of Splenda, and it just wasn't up to my expectations. A touch is inconsistent with half the speed and half the sugar.

Ingredients: for the crust

- nonstick cooking spray
- 1/2 cup chocolate graham cracker crumbs, smashed
- 1 tbsp. light butter For the filling
- 2 packets light cream cheese (8 oz.) softened
- 1/2 cup Splenda
- 1/2 cup sugar
- 1 cup canned pumpkin puree
- 3 big egg whites
- 3 tbsp. whole wheat flour
- 2 tsp. pumpkin pie spice
- 1/2 tsp. salt

Directions:

Mix the crumbs and butter in the graham cracker with the bucket until moisture is even and press into the base of the crust.

Mix the cream cheese in a stand mixer until it is creamy. Add Splenda, butter, purée of pumpkin, egg whites, rice, pumpkin pie spice, and salt. Mix once well balanced and put aside. In a safe microwave bowl, heat chocolate in 30 seconds, stirring until melted. Add 1 cup of the pumpkin mixture to the chocolate, stir and set aside. Pour the remaining pumpkin mixture into the pan and add the chocolate mixture to the pumpkin mixture. Using a knife, gently whirl the chocolate mixture through the filling to produce a marble impression. Bake for almost 40-50 minutes or until the cheese cooker is lightly tossed, but firmly threw. Cool off in the oven (I open the door) for an hour. Remove and chill, or until stiff, for at least 2 hours. Use the overhang of parchment paper, pass the cake to the work board. Using a knife soaked in sweat, break into squares, and eat.

3. DARK CHOCOLATE CHIP COCONUT COOKIES

Ingredients:

- 2 cups desiccated coconut
- 1/2 cup tapioca flour

- 1/3 cup honey
- 1 egg
- 6 tbsp. coconut oil
- 1/2 tsp. vanilla extract
- 50 g dark chocolate chunks/chips

Directions:

Preheat the oven to 180 ° C/350 ° F Temperature Combine all dry ingredients (except chocolate) in a dish. Using a blender or whisk to mix the wet ingredients, then add 4 to the dry ingredients. Mix the chocolate (you can later click the chocolate in the cookies). Shape into balls, and put on a bakery lined with six pieces of paper. Flatten balls with a fork or hand if you want a smooth cookie (sprinkle the cookies and press the dough, if you save the chocolate for now). Set in the oven for 12 minutes at 180 deg C/350 deg F or until golden brown for 8 minutes. Let the cooling rack cool and place it in an airtight jar. These cookies work even without chocolate chips. Try substituting nuts, grapes, carob, etc. 8 Ingredients Needed 25 times (minutes)

4. BLUEBERRY CRUMBLE

Delicious gluten and sugar-free alternative to the regular crumble!

Ingredients:

- 1/4 gluten-free oats (or chopped pecans / chopped walnuts if PALEO)
- 2 squash cinnamon
- 1 squash of stevia powder

- 5 squash of coconut oil (or coconut Oil if milk-free)
- 1 squash of white oats (or one squash of coconut oil if milking-free).

Directions:

Preheat the oven to 200C/400F. Place the blueberries in a cast-iron skillet. Pour the lemon juice in it and sprinkle over the berries the chia and stevia powder. Mix the almond milk, oats, cinnamon, stevia powder, and ghee in a cup. Mix the hands or a bifurcation until the ghee absorbs the "Flour." Switch the crumble to the blueberry mixture and bake for 30 minutes in the preheated oven.

Put the oven out and enjoy it!

5. JAPANESE COTTON CHEESECAKE

A delicious fluffy and spongy gluten-free and sugar-free cheesecake!

Ingredients:

- 3 eggs
- 200 g cream cheese (7 oz. * *)
- 1/2 cup white almond flour (60 g)
- 1/2 tsp. baking powder
- 1/2 tsp. stevia powder

- 1 cup blackberries (optional, I used frozen berries that I microwaved for a minute)

Directions:

Preheat in the oven to 160C/320F. Add water to the baking tray, around 2 cm, and put it on the base rack in the oven. Continue to cover the 18 cm spring bottom with a loose base. Surround the outer rim and the side of the container with the aluminum foil. Add cream to the microwave oven and microwave for forty seconds, or until smooth. Divide the eggs, put the white eggs in the bowl, and yolks in the pan with the cream cheese. While the standard cream cheese bags are 8 oz., Japanese bags are just 7 oz., so this is how I used it. I'm sure the 8 oz. pack does not make a difference, but consider adding 5-10 g of almond flour to the cake if it does.

6. KETO PUMPKIN ICE CREAM RECIPE

This milk-free ice cream is creamy, smooth, and sweet! It's the perfect treatment for fall!

Cook 5 minutes Cooling Time8 hours 25 minutes Total Time8 hours 40 minutes

NET CARBS 5.6 g

CALORIES 234kcal PROTEIN 3.22 g FAT 20.57 g

Ice Cream Maker Repo PROTEIN 3.22 g FAT 20.57 g

Ingredients:

- Ice Cream Maker Add the ice cream bowl inside the freezer overnight. Before using, make sure it's completely frozen solid. You're not supposed to hear any splashing of water inside the container.

Directions:

Add all the ingredients of the ice cream, except the egg yolks, to a medium-sized pan and place on medium heat. Whisk vigorously until the mixture begins to bubble. Turn the heat off. In a medium bowl, add the egg yolks and mix well. Add 1/4 cup (60 ml) of the hot ice cream batter to the yolks and mix well. Add another 1/4 cup and stir again. Now pour the remaining ice cream batter in the bowl and mix it all. Allow the mixture to cool down completely, about 1-2 hours, and then place in the refrigerator to cool for 2 hours. After two hours in the fridge, you will notice that the mixture of ice cream is quite thick due to coconut milk and xanthan gum.

When ready to churn, whisk back the mixture into the ice cream maker. Churn according to the manufacturer's instructions. It took 25 minutes to stir the attachment to my stand mixer. You'll have a lovely ice cream serving. Eat or move the finished ice cream into a few portions of the airtight container and put it in the freezer to cool until it is ready to serve. If you are willing to eat it, simply take it out from the refrigerator, put it 10-15 minutes down on the counter, and then enjoy it!

Please read the following tips and possible substitutions before making this recipe!

- Pre-mix the eggs in the ice cream batter. This is going to help them cook.
- Make sure to add egg yolks to the ice cream as it helps to make it smoother.
- Make sure that the ice cream batter is completely cooled in the refrigerator before adding to your ice cream maker.
- Make sure your ice cream supplier is completely frozen. You're not supposed to hear any splashing sounds from it when you take it out of the freezer.
- Use powdered erythritol to keep the grains nice and smooth. Granulated sweeteners tend to make low-carb ice creams grainy.
- Vodka is optional, but it helps to make ice cream consistent!
- You can use xylitol instead of erythritol, but do not use it if you have a dog in your house that is lethal to them.

- You can use heavy cream for the milk version instead of coconut milk.

- instead of xanthan gum, you can use guar gum.

- You can use kabocha squash purée instead of pumpkin purée.

- You can use monk fruit extract powder instead of stevia extract powder.

7. PALEO PUMPKIN PIE

The perfect milk-free pumpkin pie you'll ever produce!

Ingredients

Pie Crust:

- 280 g (9.88 oz.) white almond flour (about 2 cups thigh dessert Cuisine American, Canadian Keyword Halloween dessert, pumpkin dessert, pumpkin dessert, pumpkin pie, Thanksgiving dessert

- 280 g (9.88 oz.) white almond flour In a bowl, combine flour, lard, egg, cinnamon, and salt. Mix with a spatula until the batter sticks together and knead the hands until the ball forms.

Directions:

Wrap it with a sheet of parchment paper on the dough and cover it with a piece of paper. Roll the mixture over the paper with a rolling pin until it is a circle of around 10-11 "for a 9" glass plywood. Pel the top parchment paper and turn the dough over the 9 "pie to ensure that both sides are sealed. Peel the parchment paper and fix any problems you may have with the extra money that comes to the side. Preheat the oven to 400F/200C.In a large bowl, combine the purée of pumpkin, stevia powder, cinnamon, cloves, cardamom, ginger, and nutmeg. Mix with a whisk until it is combined. Add the coconut cream and mix again. Add the eggs one at a time while mixing until all of the batters have been added. Add the mixture to the pie plate and place in the oven. Bake for 45 minutes or so. Take it from the oven and let it cool before you serve.

- You may use almond flour for any other type of nut flour.

- You can subtract stevia from monk fruit powder to the same amount. Make sure you use a pure extract.

- You can use lard for shortening, coconut oil, beef tallow, or any other type of fat.

- You can subdue the pumpkin purée for kabocha squash, but add a little more carbs.

8. RED BERRY CLAFOUTIS

Prep period 20 mints Cook period 45 mints Overall time 1 hour 5 mints Dessert Cuisine: French Serves: 6

Ingredients:

- 1 pinch of raspberry
- 1 pinch of blueberry
- 75 g of butter
- 1 cup of plain flour

- 4 eggs
- 1/3 cup of sugar
- 1 cup of low-fat milk
- Optional: Icing sugar for dusting (for guests)

Directions:

The oven is preheated to a temperature of 180 ° C. Grease a flan dish with a little butter and starch. Shake well to distribute uniformly, then transform the dish upside down and shake once more to extract extra flour. In a single plate, apply the raspberries and blueberries to the flan. Melt the butter in a saucepan and put aside for cooling. Add rice, milk, sugar, melted butter, and combine well in a mixing pot. Heat the milk in a tiny saucepan (don't let it boil) then spill over the batter in a steady stream while you start to pound. A flat battery is going to shape. Gently spill the mixture over the fruit in the flan and bake for 45 minutes or until the surface is chocolate, Serve lukewarm or cold and icing sugar dust for your mates who are not insulin immune.

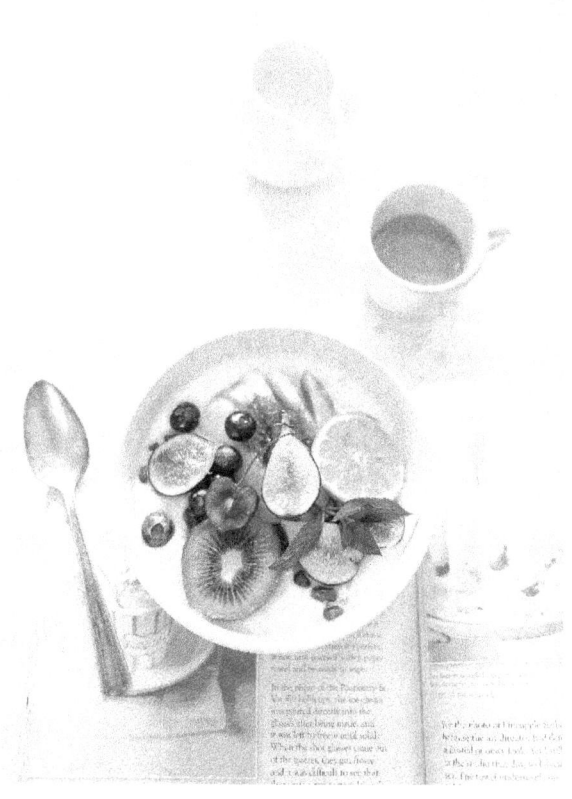

4.5 Snacks and Smoothies

1. TURMERIC TEA / GOLDEN MILK RECIPE

Drinks If you searched for natural insulin resistance supplements, you might have come across a powdered yellow spice often used in curries.

Turmeric, which has cur cumin as an active ingredient, is a magic weapon against a variety of conditions. Google the benefits of turmeric, and you will find anti-inflammatory properties, potent antioxidants, lowering blood pressure, preventing Alzheimer's, treating depression, improving brain function, reducing the risk of heart disease, (stay with me), helping with arthritis, detoxifying the liver, lowering cholesterol, preventing cancer, boosting immunity, and treating diabetes.

The "milk" in this recipe is not milk (I can't stand the taste) but coconut milk, which contains saturated fat that has been claimed to lower LDL cholesterol. To make Turmeric Tea or Golden Milk, dissolve the turmeric, cinnamon, and black pepper in coconut milk and heat the concoction.

Ingredients:

- 1/4 cup of coconut milk
- 1/4 teaspoon of turmeric
- 1/8 teaspoon of cinnamon
- 1 twist of cracked black pepper

Directions:

For a cup of coffee, add all the ingredients. Heat the microwave slowly, but don't let it bubble for 40 seconds or so. Serve in an espresso cup.

You can add hot water to the drink to make it fluffy, but I prefer it to be short to concentrate. Once you decide that your taste is excellent, a mix of spices can be made and stored in an airtight jar

2. BLACK & BLUEBERRY SMOOTHIE

Makes four servings

Ingredients:

- 2 cups of blackberries
- 2 cups of blueberries
- 1 cup of simple Greek yogurt
- 1 cup of 1 percent milk
- 1 cup of vanilla extract
- 2 cups of ice

Directions:

Layer all ingredients in a blender. Mix until nice and foamy. Serve right now.

3. ZUCCHINI CHIPS

Ingredients:

- 3-4 medium zucchini, thinly sliced
- 1 tablespoon olive oil

- Sea salt

Directions:

Cut the zucchini into thin rounds using a sharp knife or a mandolin. Place them on a paper-lined baking tray. Sprinkle with a little salt. Bake in a 160C fan for 30 minutes until it sta

4. FRUIT SALAD

Requires four servings

Ingredients:

- 1/2 cup strawberries
- 1/2 cup blueberries
- 1/2 cantaloupe
- 1/2 honeydew melon
- 1 cup seedless watermelon, cubed
- 1 mango, peeled and sliced
- 1 kiwi, peeled and sliced

Directions:

Flush the blueberries and strawberries and dump them. Remove the green tops of the strawberries cautiously and split them in two. Break the melons in half and cut the seeds. Break the melon seeds into balls or using a melon baller. Toss the cantaloupe, the honeydew melon, the watermelon, the berries, and the banana together and finish with the kiwi cut to garnish.

5. GRILLED CHICKEN AND LEMON SALAD

Are you curious about how to consume H-E-A-L-T-H-Y? Okay, chicken is still the correct option! Why? Why? Because you can't go wrong with food! Chicken, when cooked the right way and eat the right amount — that's right, no matter how good a food is, consuming too much can always make you fat — may help you lose weight! And gaining weight while you're a little above your "ideal" weight is beneficial in controlling insulin resistance — a disease under which the body's insulin responsiveness is decreased, triggering elevated blood sugar rates that can evolve into pre-diabetes or type 2 diabetes over time. Yes! Yes! So, strip the skin of your meat, roast, broil, or grill and eat!

Ingredients:

- 4 to 6 oz. skinless, boneless chicken breast
- 3/4 cup fresh lemon juice
- 1/4 cup olive oil
- 1 tablespoon fresh thyme leaves
- 1 teaspoon salt

- 1 cup chopped sugar peas
- 1/2 cup red bell pepper, strips
- 1/2 cup yellow bell pepper, strips

Directions:

Put the chicken inside the bag and then close it. Place in the refrigerator and marinate for one hour, turning periodically. After marinating, remove the marinade and place the chicken on a grill rack filled with a cooking mist. Grill on each hand for about 6 minutes. Split the grilled chicken into 1/4-inch thick slices. Set it aside. Carry the water to a boil and cook the sweet peas for around 30 seconds. Drain, then spray with fresh water. In a big pot, mix the cooked sugar with the red and yellow bell pepper, the zucchini strips, the minced fresh cilantro, the extra virgin olive oil, the salt, and the ground black pepper. Add some chicken. Flip to be mixed. Serve with a lemon wedge and enjoy!

6. CHOCOLATE CHERRY CINNAMON SMOOTHIE

Ingredients:

- 1 1/2 x cups of fresh or frozen cherries (if frozen, add sugar)
- 1 x banana
- 1/2 x cup of coconut milk

- 2 x tbsp. Sweetened cocoa powder
- 2 x tsp. Cinnamon
- 3/4 cup water
- 4 x ice cubes

Directions:

Mix all ingredients until they are smooth and enjoyable!

This diet is low in sodium and cholesterol. It is an excellent source of copper and dietary fiber and an excellent source of manganese.

Fill the mixer with all the ingredients. Mix until smooth. Mix until smooth. Add additional water if necessary until the desired consistency is achieved. Split evenly among two large glasses and enjoy!

This diet is low in sodium and cholesterol. This is also a good source of vitamin C and manganese. This is also anti-inflammatory STRONGLY.

7. TOMATO & MOZZARELLA POCKETS

Ingredients:

- 2 whole wheat pita bread squares, sliced in half to produce four pockets
- 2 ripe tomatoes, chopped

- 4 teaspoons of olive oil

- 4 (1 ounce) slices of part-skim mozzarella cheese

- 1 garlic clove, chopped

- 1 cup of fresh basil leaves, chopped

- Salt and pepper

Directions:

Warm up the pockets of the pita. Place the tomatoes, mozzarella, garlic, and basil in a cup, sprinkle with salt and pepper to compare and drizzle with olive oil. Layer all ingredients in the pita bags.

8. MIXED BERRY SMOOTHIE

Ingredients:

- 100ml (1/2 cup) x Almond Milk

- 1 x Medium Banana

- 80 g (3 oz.) x Frozen Mixed Berries

- 1 x Spinach

- 1 x Hemp or Pea Protein

- Water as required

Directions:

In a juicer, place all the ingredients and combine them until they are smooth. If your smoothie is too thick, add water until the desired consistency is achieved.

9. SUGAR-FREE LEMONADE

Beat your sugar cravings with this simple, lemonade!

Prep Time 5 minutes Total Time 5 minutes

SERVICES PEOPLE

NET CARBS1.57 g CALORIES5kcal PROTEIN0.07 g

INGREDIENTS:

- 5 tbsp. of lemon juice (from real lemons is better)
- 1000 mL cold water
- 1/8 tsp. stevia powder

Directions:

Wash your lemons' skin. Squeeze the juice out of your fruits with a lemon squeezer until you have about 5 tbsp. Reject the seeds. Slice the remaining fruit into thick slices. Connect the big container with lemon juice, water, and stevia powder. Shake well, dude. Shake well. Attach the slices of lemon to the bowl. If you want to, eat cold with some ice cubes.

10. COCONUT OIL AND PCOS

Coconut and palm oil have received a lot of coverage in recent years. It's expected to be a perfect oil that can cope with being fried at high temperatures and has excellent antimicrobial properties.

Although, when it comes to PCOS, there are many advantages to coconut oil.

Waist circumference Work has shown that coconut oil can help boost metabolism and help the waist circumference.

Women with PCOS continue to gain weight around their waist (in reality, our abdominal fat cells are more significant than average, allowing us to gain weight around our waist and abdomen).

As a consequence, coconut oil will help combat some of this buildup of fat around the heart.

Inflammation, the added advantage of coconut oil is that it assists reduce inflammation. People who use coconut oil instead of other vegetable oils appear to have lower rates of oxidative stress and inflammatory markers. People with PCOS are now vulnerable to inflammation. The swelling also renders us more prone to insulin, giving our PCOS worse. So, we need to do what we can to control our degree of inflammation.

A word of caution Before we go-to coconut oil, we need to be careful. One teaspoon of coconut oil produces 130 calories. It's crucial to keep that in mind, particularly if you're trying to lose weight.

Ingredients:

- 1 x cup of shredded / deserted coconut
- 4 x tablespoons of coconut oil (melted or runny)
- 1/4 x cup of honey
- 1 x cup of vanilla essence

Directions:

Mix all the components in a mixing pot. Place the mixture in a small flat bowl. Refrigerate for an hour or two. Split it to offer. Place in the refrigerator in an airtight jar.

11. THE NOT-SO BLOODY MARY

Let's face her. There are times when you need a kick to start your morning, and a cup of coffee alone won't do that. Enter the Bloody Mary with all her liquor, spice, and warm glory to give a much-needed kick to your head.

Tomato juice is on the authorized list of what to eat on the insulin resistance diet – albeit in small quantities. Always choose tomato juice with no added sugar. It tastes better for a start, and you won't feel guilty for enjoying it. Bloody Mary is a delicious drink, and there are enough natural sugars and carbs in tomatoes that you don't need anymore.

Ingredients:

- 200 ml of tomato juice (no added sugar)
- 1 teaspoon of Worcestershire sauce
- 2-3 tablespoons of Tabasco sauce
- Sprinkles of celery salt
- Squeeze of lemon
- Optional: Celery stick or asparagus for garnish

Directions:

In a glass, pour all the ingredients and stir. Serve with a celery stick or asparagus for garnish.

CONCLUSION

The one phrase that most stresses in these research papers are insulin resistance. Insulin and insulin resistance tend to be the most prominent cause of PCOS. This suggests that it is better to place someone with PCOS in a diet that will reduce insulin rates and decrease insulin resistance, as in the case of a ketogenic diet.

Before we come to any conclusions, we do need to remember the PCOS legacy reports. In the studies, this condition has an independent genetic effect on the lifestyle factor, which raises the question — are PCOS-induced women?

Many researchers believe that genetic variations lead to PCOS. For instance, a recent study by Miller and colleagues found that PCOS and insulin resistance may be associated with a single genetic defect. The second group of researchers proposed that fetal modifications cause the genetic defect(s) leading to PCOS. In other words, if the fetus develops in the mother when she is in a stressful environment (i.e., without sufficient nourishment), then genetic modifications are made to make the fetus adapt to the stressful setting.

One of these genetic adaptations is resistance to insulin. While PCOS, heart disease, obesity, and diabetes type 2 are associated with insulin resistance, they are helpful when food is scarce as energy is stored in the blood for a longer time so that it can enter the cells that most need it. However, many of us live in food productive climates. Chips, cakes, or any other food you like will influence your taste buds in around 30 minutes. This combination of resistance to insulin and the intake of excess calories is a formula for chronic diseases.

But thinking precisely what does this have to do with PCOS women? Scientists claim that certain women develop a particular form of insulin resistance that shuts off their reproductive cycle and raises their testosterone levels so that they have an increased chance of survival. It can, however, only cause PCOS symptoms if the woman is excessively depressed, or sedentary.

PCOS genes are inheritable, but they don't mean you're infertile. Later, we will learn how fertility is triggered (and PCOS removed), but first, let us understand how PCOS is made. The scientific literature on PCOS diets is sparse. But the therapy analysis researchers say that PCOS women will do better to eat complex carbohydrates and avoid sugar. This suggestion has been confirmed in one study on the impact of the low-glycemic index diet on women with PCOS, but the findings of related research on the ketogenic diet are unimpressive.

Five overweight women eat a ketogenic diet for 24 weeks (20 grams or less of carbohydrates a day). The findings were remarkable – an average weight loss of 12%, free testosterone decreased by 22%, and fasting insulin concentrations decreased by 54%. Perhaps more impressive is that amid prior infertility issues, two of the women became pregnant.

This provides experimental proof of the efficacy of the ketogenic diet for PCOS treatment. This result, however, is not shocking. Ketogenic diets have been shown to raise insulin levels and minimize insulin resistance in several different groups of people, from safe subjects to Type 2 diabetic patients — two factors which would also benefit women PCOS. Ketogenic diets also result in rapid loss of weight, which in obese women with PCOS is essential to enhance fertility.

There is, therefore, significant protection for women and the ketogenic diet. Restricting carbohydrates in the ketogenic diet can lead to increased stress and resistance to insulin. Thus, the ketogenic diet should be followed, with slight modifications, if appropriate. Many women will reverse their PCOS with a pure ketogenic diet. However, for some women, the reduction in carbohydrates can cause unnecessary stress and prevent performance. Therefore, following these guidelines to build the right PCOS diet for you is crucial:

Restrict carbohydrates It is suggested to start with less than 35 g total carbohydrates per day. If you get worse with symptoms a few weeks later, increasing your intake of carbohydrates by 5-10 grams a day before you reach a sweet spot where you feel better. Seek to reduce your consumption by 5-10 grams a day from your current intake level to increase your ketone level and fat-burning ability. Eat high fiber vegetables with any food. High fiber vegetables, such as broccoli and spinach, can help resist insulin and reduce inflammation. Have them for better results with every meal. See our low-carbon vegetable guide for more about what to eat and how to add to your diet. Using our keto calculator to find out what your average intake of protein will be. Use our calculator to estimate your average daily calorie intake, eat enough calories to reach your ideal weight again. If your body fat level is unhealthily low, make sure you have more calories to consume than you need to maintain your weight. You must manage a calorie deficit to lose weight if you are overweight or obese.

You can reduce your insulin levels, regulate your hormones, and reverse many of the PCOS symptoms by following these guidelines. Nevertheless, tension and inactivity will still restrict the outcomes. Combine a balanced lifestyle with a ketogenic diet to produce the best results.

Polycystic ovary syndrome (PCOS) accounts for up to 70 percent of women's infertility problems. Also, it causes symptoms such as acne, male shallowness, mood swings, weight gain, and fatigue, making it a painful condition. Fortunately, with the proper combination of diet, workout, sleep, and meditation, you can reverse PCOS. For instance, the ketogenic diet may be one of the best foods for PCOS women since insulin levels and insulin resistance is decreased.

It is highly probable that you combine a ketogenic diet with 30 minutes of daily exercise, 7-9 hours of quality sleep and daily meditation with PCOS. You can use various supplements to support you with the new diet and lifestyle. By supplementing extra starch and by taking magnesium and Rishi mushrooms in limited doses, pressures that may make PCOS worse can be alleviated. Certain natural dietary supplements, such as inositol, calcium, apple vinegar, cinnamon, flaxseeds, and bebeerine, can improve health and PCOS symptoms more quickly. Make sure you consult your doctor in the process of reversing PCOS. He/she can order various blood tests to confirm how well your new diet and lifestyle work for you.

www.ingramcontent.com/pod-product-compliance
Lightning Source LLC
Chambersburg PA
CBHW052351220526
45465CB00003BA/1063